THE COMFORT CRISIS

EMBRACE DISCOMFORT

TO RECLAIM YOUR

WILD, HAPPY, HEALTHY SELF

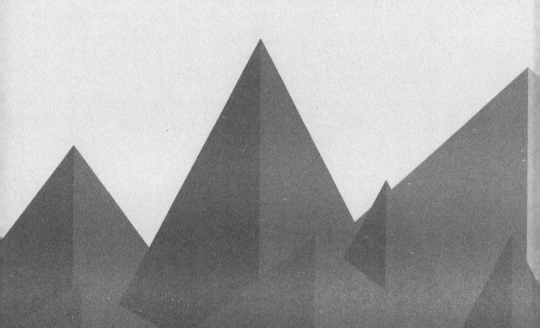

THE
COMFORT
CRISIS

MICHAEL EASTER

RODALE BOOKS
NEW YORK

rodalebooks.com

RODALE and the Plant colophon are registered trademarks of
Penguin Random House LLC.

Library of Congress Cataloging-in-Publication Data
is available upon request.

ISBN 978-0-593-13876-2
Ebook ISBN 978-0-593-13877-9

Printed in the United States of America

Book design by Jen Valero
Jacket design by Pete Garceau
Jacket photo-illustration by
bgblue/DigitalVision Vectors/Getty Images (door) and
hadynyah/E+/Getty Images (landscape)

10 9 8 7 6 5 4 3 2 1

First Edition

To Leah, who always makes me laugh and never bullshits me

CONTENTS

PART ONE
Rule 1: Make it really hard. Rule 2: Don't die.

PART TWO
Rediscover boredom. Ideally outside. For minutes, hours, and days.

PART THREE
Feel hunger.

PART FOUR
Think about your death every day.

PART FIVE
Carry the load.

PART ONE

Rule 1: Make it really hard.

Rule 2: Don't die.

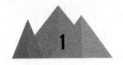

33 DAYS

I'M STANDING ON a windy tarmac in Kotzebue, Alaska, a 3,000-person village 20 miles above the Arctic Circle on the Chukchi Sea. In front of me are two airplanes. One will soon dump me deep into the Alaskan Arctic, a place that's generally agreed to be one of the loneliest, most remote, and most hostile on earth. I'm on edge.

This impending voyage into the Arctic is one thing. But I'm also no fan of flying. Particularly when it's in planes like these: single-engine, two- and four-seater bush craft. Picture empty Campbell's soup cans with wings.

Donnie Vincent senses my nerves. He's a backcountry bow-hunter and documentary filmmaker on this expedition with me. He sidles up to my shoulder, leans in, and lowers his voice. "Most of the pilots up here are whiskey-swilling cowboy mountain men. The type of guys who don't think twice about getting into a bar fight," he says over the freezing gusts. "But just so you know, I booked the absolute best pilot I could. Brian is Top Gun." I nod thanks.

"I'm not telling you we're *not* going to crash and die," Donnie continues. "That is a real risk, OK? But this guy is good. So the odds that we'll be in a plane crash are . . ." My edginess amplifies into existential dread as I cut him off. "OK," I say. "Got it."

Commercial flying is incredibly safe. The statistics say you're infinitely more likely to die in a crash on the way to the airport than you are in the plane. But this rule does not apply to bush plane flights in Alaska.

About 100 of these flights a year end in fire and brimstone, and the FAA recently released an "unprecedented warning" to Alaskan bush plane pilots after a spike in accidents. This year has been particularly bad. Fierce weather and thick fog and wildfire smoke have been messing with visibility. Donnie tells me that Brian has a colleague named Mike who recently crashed after misreading the weather. Mike was lucky enough to walk away, but the plane had to be rebuilt.

Once Brian drops us in the Arctic backcountry, we'll face more dangers: furious grizzlies, 1,500-pound moose, packs of flesh-craving wolves, wild-eyed wolverines, blood-addicted badgers, raging glacial rivers, violent whiteout snowstorms, subzero temperatures, hurricane-force winds, precipitous cliffs, deadly diseases with names like tularemia and hantavirus, swarming mosquitoes, swarming mice, swarming rats, the runs, the barfs, the bleeds. . . . There might be a million ways to die in the West, but there are 2 million in the Alaskan backcountry.

Our only way out? We'll trudge hundreds of miles across that rugged world until Brian picks us up in 33 days' time. Along the way we'll be searching for a mythical herd of caribou, a migrating army of 400-pound ghosts that silently roam the Arctic tundra, their gnarled, four-foot antlers emerging from the crystalline fog only to disappear when the wind shifts.

The coming five weeks are an all-in proposition. Unlike, say, hiking the Pacific Crest or the Appalachian Trail, deep in the Alaskan backcountry you can't decide you're too cold and hungry and wander a couple miles off-trail to a highway where you can Uber to the nearest diner for a hot cup of coffee and a stack of flapjacks. There are few, if any, trails. And the closest road, town, point of cell reception, and hospital can be hundreds of miles away. Hell, even death may not be a way out. My insurance policy, unfortunately, does not offer "remotely located corpse recovery" coverage.

None of this sounds anything like my safe, comfortable life at home. And that's the point. Most people today rarely step outside their comfort zones. We are living progressively sheltered, sterile, temperature-controlled, overfed, underchallenged, safety-netted lives. And it's limiting the degree to which we experience our "one wild and precious life," as poet Mary Oliver put it.

But a radical new body of evidence shows that people are at their best—physically harder, mentally tougher, and spiritually sounder—after experiencing the same discomforts our early ancestors were exposed to every day. Scientists are finding that certain discomforts protect us from physical and psychological problems like obesity, heart disease, cancers, diabetes, depression, and anxiety, and even more fundamental issues like feeling a lack of meaning and purpose.

There are plenty of, let's say, less committed ways to gain the benefits of discomfort. Stuff a person could easily fold into their daily life to improve their mind, body, and spirit. But this trip is at the extreme end of a prescription that researchers across disciplines say we should make a part of our lives. It's part rewilding, part rewiring. And its benefits are all-encompassing.

Brian, Donnie, William Altman, who is Donnie's lifelong cinematographer, and I are outside the Conex shipping container that acts as Ram Aviation's base of operations at Kotzebue's local airport. We're all organizing gear and trying to keep our faces out of the ballistic wind, which is shuttling more salty fog from the sea across the land and into the hazy gray mountains. "Let's load up and go before that fog gets worse," says Brian.

Donnie used to spend six months at a time in the Alaskan backcountry as a biologist for the Fish and Wildlife Service. He lived out of a yellow North Face tent that he describes as a "big yellow gumdrop." He's since researched, hunted, and filmed in some of the most extreme and remote locations on earth. The guy one summer, no kidding, lived among a pack of wolves as he studied salmon on the Tuluksak River in the Yukon delta.

William has been with Donnie on nearly every hunt and is a rare breed of twenty-something who parties like it's 1899. He spent most of the last decade in an Internet- and running-water-free, eight-foot-by-eight-foot cabin in the Maine backwoods. The kid primarily lives on food he hunts, raises, and grows himself.

The accompaniment of these guys eases my apprehension. But only sort of. Because the thing about nature is that it's unpredictable and unforgiving. It doesn't care about your experience and what happened the last time you visited it. Nature can always throw rougher stuff at you. Meaner animals, taller cliffs, lower temperatures, wider rivers, and more snow, rain, wind, and sleet.

Donnie and William are often reminded of this harrowing reality. They once ran out of food and nearly starved and froze when whiteout storms caused their pickup plane to arrive four days late. Another time they had to shoot a charging locomotive-size grizzly that would have rearranged their internal organs. By dumb luck the shot ricocheted off the bear's skull, knocking him out cold.

I grab my 80-pound backpack, which carries most everything I'll need to survive over the next month. Layers of clothing, food, emergency medical kit, etc. Brian stops me as I'm lugging the bag over to his plane.

"You and William are in that one," he says, pointing to a freshly painted green-and-gold four-seater Cessna. We muscle our packs into the plane's hull, and I step up into its passenger door and contort myself into its backseat. My knees are jammed up into my throat back here.

Donnie and Brian hop into the other plane. It circles the runway and takes off toward the fog as William and I sit waiting in the Cessna. And here comes our pilot. He's young, with a ball cap over a high and tight haircut. Aviator sunglasses. He struts up and slithers into the pilot's seat. Reaches out a gloved hand for a shake.

"Hi," he says. "I'm your pilot, Mike."

William peers back at me with a twisted grin. *Wait,* I think, *is this the same Mike that crashed his plane?* The propeller kicks, stoking decibels that drown out my inner scream.

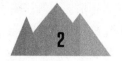

35, 55, OR 75

I COME FROM a long line of men who seem to run on booze, bullshit, and self-serving chaos. My father, who disappeared while I was in the womb, once got drunk on St. Patrick's Day, painted his horse green, and rode it into a bar with a woman who was not my mother. An uncle once spent a night in a dry-out cell screaming, for reasons unknown to him and everyone in that particular correctional facility on that particular Tuesday night, "Your. Mom. Fucks. Volkswagens!" A cousin once came to in the county jail and found that he'd blacked out into an impromptu family reunion—the police had thrown him into a cell with one of my uncles. Yet another uncle is a frequent drop-in at the Idaho state prison. And my grandfather was roundly agreed to be the most charming and handsome liar, cheat, and drunk in Ada County.

Nearly a decade ago, I found myself riding that same family horse. There were a couple of "Dude, where's my car?" moments, some broken bones and bent relationships, and I was once arrested during an intoxicated attempt to break the land-speed record on a collapsible scooter.

I was also something of a professional hypocrite. I had an enviable career at a glossy magazine as a health journalist dispensing advice on how to live a better life. I was good at the job. But I wasn't exactly living the wisdom I wrote. Most of my mental energy was spent toggling back and forth between being drunk and obsessing over the next drink.

Nearly everything in my life deferred to alcohol. If I wasn't drinking, I was running out the clock until the weekend, when I'd drink again. This practice made my life a fast-moving fog, and I lost years in a cycle of weekend bingeing. I'd march Monday to Friday from hangover to swearing off booze to recovery to convincing myself that this time it would be different to being shitfaced again.

Alcohol was my comfort blanket. It killed the stress around my job. It quickly ended boredom. It numbed me to sadness, anxiety, and fear. It covered me from what was uncomfortable: the insecurities, situations, thoughts, and emotions that are just part of being a human.

Then, at 28, I awoke one morning soaked in misery and whiskey-tinged vomit. It was the second morning like that in a row, and I'd had plenty like it before. But this time around I experienced one of those moments I didn't understand at the time, except that I knew something big was happening.

I experienced clarity, a state that was at the time about as familiar to me as particle physics. I could see my life as it was and not as I believed it to be. I was a tongue-chewing idiot drunk and career fraud, and everything around me was a damn mess that was only getting messier with each ensuing weekend.

I could see that I'd soon be found out and lose my job. Next would be my relationships, because being around me while I was drinking was fun until it wasn't, which usually occurred sometime after the fifth drink. Then would go my possessions. Car, house, etc. Eventually I'd lose my life. Whether I'd die at 35, 55, or 75, I didn't know. I just knew that my drinking habit was going to end me early. People who say things like "Let's finish these beers and then ride those ATVs" aren't exactly models of longevity. Comfort from alcohol was not only numbing me to the life I wanted to live, it was also killing me.

I saw a choice. Option one, do nothing. Cling to complacency and the numbing lifestyle that would ultimately end badly but allow me to keep drinking. All evidence until then suggested that nothing fixes a problem like the first drink.

Or option two, get uncomfortable. Ditch my liquid comfort blanket. I hadn't a clue where this second route would take me or if I could even pull it off. And I was terrified. But the funny thing about waking up covered in your own stomach contents is that it makes doing the exact opposite of whatever got you there an easier decision to make. No one gets sober on a Friday evening. It's a Sunday-morning-coming-down kind of a decision.

I raised the white flag. This is when the discomfort started.

The acute physical hell of drying out lasted for days. There were headaches, nausea, exhaustion, the shakes, the sweats, and other internal hells. My lungs began kicking up what I can only imagine was some kind of a carcinogen cocktail, because I had a habit of chasing drinks with Marlboros.

The physical stuff eventually faded below the line of perception. But then the even bigger challenge of sobriety started—dealing with my frenetic thoughts as my booze-altered brain began to rewire itself. My mind was like a hard rubber ball shot from a cannon into a concrete room. It existed in a high-grade state of mania and bounced from joy that I was alive, to depression that I got here, to terrifying question after terrifying question about my new way of life. How do I not drink? What do I do on weekends? What should I say if I'm at a social event and someone asks me if I want a drink? How will I reconnect with my old friends at college reunions and weddings?

It turns out the answers to those questions are: "Don't drink," "Anything but drinking," "No, thanks," and "Why don't you cross that bridge when you come to it, bud?" I understand the simplicity now. But at the time these were profound, baffling questions, like asking a toddler to solve for x. It comes as no shock to me that half of people admitted to mental health institutions suffer from substance abuse disorders. I required a relearning of life and how to live it.

And there were generations of whiskey-bent, hell-bound Easter family chromosomes fighting this new path. These types of genes are coded to make you believe that The Solution is a smoky barroom with a jukebox that plays George Jones, and that things will go right this round despite hundreds of examples of evidence to the contrary.

But day by day I embraced the raw discomfort of hard change, and soon the world opened up. I became aware of the beauty of being alive and better understood my role. Before sobriety, for example, all signs seemed to indicate that I was the absolute center of the universe. But upon drying out I realized that I'm just not that damn important in the grand scheme of things. This is a deeply unnerving recognition. But once I started to act on it—admitting that I don't know things and that I could use some help—I gained some peace and perspective.

I began connecting with the people I love in new, deeper ways. I started to find silence, experience calm, and feel OK with myself. To get out of myself, I got a dog and each morning took him to a nearby river, where I felt a long-forgotten peace and confidence in the 5 a.m. quiet and mist. I became less flustered by everyday problems like work dramas, traffic jams, deadlines, and bills.

I wasn't a completely new person and I'd never be confused with Mr. Rogers. But I was more aware, which allowed me to see that I was still surrounded in comfort. I was marinating in the stuff. Except that these were less acutely destructive but potentially more insidious forms of it. I just had to take a look at my everyday life. I was comfortable, quite literally, every single moment.

I awoke in a soft bed in a temperature-controlled home. I commuted to work in a pickup with all the conveniences of a luxury sedan. I killed any semblance of boredom with my smartphone. I sat in an ergonomic desk chair staring at a screen all day, working with my mind and not my body. When I arrived home from work, I filled my face with no-effort, highly caloric foods that came from Lord knows where. Then I plopped down on my overstuffed sofa to binge on television streamed down from outer space. I rarely, if ever, felt the sensation of discomfort. The most physically uncomfortable thing I did, exercise, was executed inside an air-conditioned building as I watched cable news channels that are increasingly bent on confirming my worldview rather than challenging it. I wouldn't run outside unless the conditions were, well, comfortable. Neither too hot, too cold, nor too wet.

What could cleansing myself of all these other comforts do for me?

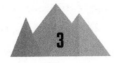

0.004 PERCENT

HUMANS EVOLVED TO seek comfort. We instinctually default to safety, shelter, warmth, extra food, and minimal effort. And that drive through nearly all of human history was beneficial because it pushed us to survive.

Discomfort is both physical and emotional. It's hunger, cold, pain, exhaustion, stress, and any other trying sensations and emotions. Our comfort drive led us to find food. To build and take shelter. To flee from predators. To avoid overly risky decisions. To do anything and everything that would help us live on and spread our DNA. So it's really no surprise that today we should still default to that which is most comfortable.

Except that our original comforts were negligible and short-lived, at best. In an uncomfortable world, consistently seeking a sliver of comfort helped us stay alive. Our common problem today is that our environment has changed, but our wiring hasn't. And this wiring is deeply ingrained.

About 2.5 million years ago, our ancestor *Homo habilis* evolved out of the smartest apelike animals of the time. These men and women walked on two feet and used stone tools, giving them an edge in the wild. But they didn't look much like us (picture a chimp crossed with a modern human), and their brain was about half the size of ours.

Then, 1.8 million years ago, came *Homo erectus.* This species looked and behaved more like us. They stood about five foot ten and lived in social hunter-gatherer societies. They likely figured out how to use fire, and thought abstractly, which we surmise because they created art by engraving designs into objects they found in nature. Sure, this art was more spastic two-year-old than Sistine Chapel, but progress is progress.

Next, about 700,000 years ago, came *Homo heidelbergensis* and then *Homo neanderthalensis.* Their brains were actually slightly larger than ours and they'd picked up all the skills from their predecessors, like using tools, creating fire, and more. They also learned to build homes, make clothes, and—consequentially—master hunting. They were apex predators. Using stone-tipped spears, they'd take down animals like red deer, rhinoceroses, and even mammoths. The now extinct, massively trunked mammoth could weigh as much as a Kenworth semitruck.

Despite what insurance advertisements will have us believe, *Homo heidelbergensis* and *neanderthalensis* were not idiots. Their epic hunts required coordinated teamwork. A single man or woman against a mammoth is a massacre for that man or woman. But with *men and women*—a team of them strategizing and working together—we did damage. This is when our ancestors began to understand that putting our heads together to solve common problems could help us not only survive but also live a little better.

Which brings us to us. Our species, called *Homo sapiens,* has been walking this earth for 200,000 to 300,000 years, depending on which anthropologist you ask. And we are highly evolved, despite what you may see on reality TV like *Cops* or any of the *Housewives* franchises. Early *Homo sapiens* developed complex tools, languages, cities, currency, farming, transportation systems, and much more. And that was before all of the human history we have written down, which is only about 5,000 years' worth of time.

The modern comforts and conveniences that now most influence our daily experience—cars, computers, television, climate control, smartphones, ultraprocessed food, and more—have been used by our species for about 100 years or less. That's around 0.03 percent of the time we've walked the earth. Include all the *Homos*—*habilis, erectus, heidelbergensis, neanderthalensis,* and us—and open the time scale to 2.5 million years and the figure drops to 0.004 percent. Constant comfort is a radically new thing for us humans.

Over these 2.5 million years, our ancestors' lives were intimately intertwined with discomfort. These people were constantly exposed to the elements. It was either too hot, too cold, too wet, too dry, too windy, or too snowy out. The only escape from the weather was a rudimentary shelter, like a cold, damp cave filled with bats and rats, or a hole dug in the ground and roofed with twigs or an animal skin. Or some other crude structure that provided enough shelter to keep a person alive but little else. Today most of us live at 72 degrees, experiencing weather only during the two minutes it takes us to walk across a parking lot or from the subway station to our offices. Americans now spend about 93 percent of our time indoors in climate control, and entire cities wouldn't exist had we not developed air-conditioning. Like Phoenix and Las Vegas.

Early humans were always hungry. The Hadza, a Tanzanian tribe of hunter-gatherers that lives similarly to our earliest ancestors, are constantly complaining to anthropologists that they're ravenous. And not the kind of mindless hunger that comes from watching the Food Network. They experience deep, persistent hunger.

Early humans surely did not have constant, effortless access to calorie-dense food. They either had to walk miles to find the right place to dig it deep out of the ground or pick it high off a tree. Or they had to face off with animals both tiny and towering. The Hadza are to this day constantly being stung by swarms of bees when they gather honey, a delicacy for the tribe. Nearly 80 percent of Neanderthals' bones show signs that their owner had either been maimed or outright killed by animals. Now we can order delivery through an app or drop by a Super Walmart and buy anything and everything—from honey in a cute plastic bear container to meats packaged in plastic wrap—and be rather confident that our errand will not end in grievous bodily harm.

When our ancestors weren't searching for food or getting pummeled by mastodons, they had long moments of downtime, lounging around for hours a day. They had to make something out of their boredom.

These people allowed their minds to wander and had to get creative and rely on one another for entertainment. As my beautifully blunt then-girlfriend, now-wife put it when we went camping early in our relationship: "We ran out of things to talk about in three hours and had a whole day left." It wasn't until the 1920s, when radio was broadcast to the masses, that there was a full-time, brainless escape from boredom. Then came Big TV in the 1950s. Finally, on June 29, 2007, boredom was pronounced dead, thanks to the iPhone. And so our imaginations and deep social connections went with it.

When they weren't sitting and doing nothing, our ancestors were working very, very hard. The Hadza exercise 14 times more than the average American. They move fast and hard about 2 hours and 20 minutes a day. (Although, to be clear, what they're doing is just called "life" instead of "exercise.") Early humans would walk or run miles and miles for water and food. In fact, the reason the human body is built the way it is—with arched feet, long leg tendons, sweat glands, and more—is because we evolved to run down prey. We'd chase and track the animal for miles and miles until it toppled over from heat exhaustion. Then we'd kill it, butcher it, and carry it all the way back to camp. When prey was too heavy to haul, our ancestors would pick up camp and move to the downed food.

They faced stress. Lots of it. If they didn't find food, they died. If a lion decided he wanted their food, they died (or ran, or got mauled). If they got too far away from water, they died. If violent weather hit, they died. If they got an infection, they died. If they tripped and fractured a leg, they died. And on and on.

Sure, modern humans are stressed. More stressed than ever before, according to the American Psychological Association. But we don't suffer from the type of acute stresses humans fretted over for millions of years. Most of us don't experience physical stresses like feeling intense hunger, exhaustion from running down food, carrying heavy loads, or exposing ourselves to freak germs and wild temperature swings. Nor do we suffer from mental stresses like wondering where our next meal is coming from, fearing fanged predators, or dreading that a little nick could get infected and kill us off in a week. The Covid-19 pandemic, in fact, was likely the first time that many of us felt our forgotten stresses and realized that humans can still be powerless against the natural world.

For most modern Americans, "stress" is so often "This traffic is going to make me late to my yoga class" stress. Or "Is my neighbor making more money than me?" stress. Or "This spreadsheet is going to take forever" stress. Or "If my child doesn't get into an Ivy League school we will all live lives of complete and utter nothingness" stress. It's first-world stress.

This is why many scholars have written about how the world is, as a whole, improving. They point out that people are living longer and better, are making more money, and are less likely to be murdered or go hungry than at any time before. Even the poorest Americans are well off relative to the grand sweep of generations before them. And yes, many numbers and data and graphs do indeed suggest that the world is better. Of course the world is better!

But there's a catch: Because our ancestors dealt with so much discomfort, there were many things they *didn't* have to deal with. Namely, the most pressing problems that modern cultures are facing right now. Problems that are making many of our lives unhealthier, unhappier, and less than they could be.

Thanks to modern medicine the average person is, yes, living longer than ever. But the data shows that the majority of us are living a greater proportion of our years in ill health, propped up by medications and machines. Life span might be up. But health span is down.

Thirty-two percent of Americans are overweight and 38 percent are obese. Eight percent of the latter classify as "extremely obese." That makes a collective 70 percent of us too heavy. Nearly a third of us now have diabetes or prediabetes. More than 40 million Americans have mobility problems that hinder them from getting from point A to B. Heart disease kills a quarter of us. These are all medical issues that were essentially nonexistent until the twentieth century.

People today are also suffering more and more from diseases of despair: depression, anxiety, addiction, and suicide. Overdose deaths in the last two decades are up more than threefold, and the average American is now more likely to kill themselves than ever before. Evidence suggests that suicide didn't happen throughout nearly all of human history. My high school graduating class of 400, for example, has lost anywhere from 1 to 3 people each year to overdoses or suicides since we earned our diplomas.

These diseases of despair caused the US life expectancy to fall in 2016, 2017, and 2018. There hasn't been a life span drop like this since the period from 1915 to 1918, when World War I and the Spanish Flu pandemic united in a symphony of death.

So, yes, we don't have to deal with discomforts like working for our food, moving hard and heavy each day, feeling deep hunger, and being exposed to the elements. But we do have to deal with the side effects of our comfort: long-term physical and mental health problems.

We lack physical struggles, like having to work hard for our livelihoods. We have too many ways to numb out, like comfort food, cigarettes, alcohol, pills, smartphones, and TV. We're detached from the things that make us feel happy and alive, like connection, being in the natural world, effort, and perseverance.

We seem to know *something* is amiss. One poll found just 6 percent of Americans believe the world is improving. Some anthropologists, in fact, argue that humans were happier in all the time leading up to about 13,000 years ago. People then had simpler needs that were easier to fulfill and were more able to live in the present.

Comforts and conveniences are great. But they haven't always moved the ball downfield in our most important metric: happy, healthful years. Perhaps existing *only* in our increasingly overly comfortable, overbuilt environment and *always* obeying our comfort drives has had unintended consequences and caused us to miss profound human experiences. There are conditions that humans evolved to live in and experiences we were meant to have that are no longer germane to our lives. This has undoubtedly changed us, often not for the best.

800 FACES

DAVID LEVARI IS in his early 30s and a psychologist at Harvard University. He's the picture of an up-and-coming Ivy League doctor of psychology: impeccably spoken, perfectly bearded, and interested in investigating big questions about why humans behave the way we do.

Levari was studying under the famed researcher Dan Gilbert when the two were traveling to a conference. As they stood in line for airport security, they noticed something funny. The TSA agents treat a lot of clearly nonthreatening people like existential risks.

We've all experienced the phenomenon in real life. Some well-meaning TSA agent rips apart a carry-on seemingly thinking someone's banana is a 9mm Beretta. Or a wheelchair-bound 90-year-old who can't walk or see gets the full-body pat-down after forgetting she had a half-full bottle of hairspray in her purse.

Obviously the phrase *better safe than sorry* applies here. "But we wondered," said Levari, "if all of a sudden people stopped bringing stuff that wasn't allowed into the airport and the luggage scanners never went off, would the TSA just relax and do nothing?" They didn't think so. "Our intuition was that the TSA would do what most of us would do," he said. "When they ran out of stuff to find they would start looking for a wider range of stuff, even if this was not conscious or intentional, because their job is to look for threats."

With that in mind, Levari recently conducted a series of studies to find out if the human brain searches for problems even when problems become infrequent or don't exist. One of his studies tasked people with viewing a sequence of 800 different human faces that ranged from very intimidating to completely harmless.

The people had to judge which of the faces seemed "threatening." But once they'd seen the 200th mug, Levari (without the participants' knowledge) began showing them fewer and fewer "threatening faces."

Another of Levari's studies used a similar setup. Except this time the people were asked to deem whether 240 scientific research proposals were "ethical" or "unethical." About midway through, Levari began giving the people successively fewer "unethical" proposals.

These two scenarios should be rather black-and-white, right? A person is either threatening or not. A proposal either does or does not cross a moral line. Because if we can't see these situations as black-and-white, then it calls into question whether we can really trust our judgment in much bigger issues. Like, it turns out, just how comfortable we've become and how that's affecting us.

When he looked at all the data, Levari discovered that humans can't see black or white. We see gray. And the shade of gray we see depends on all of the other shades that came before it. We adjust expectations.

As the threatening faces became rare, the study participants began to perceive neutral faces as threatening. When the unethical research proposals became less frequent, people began deeming ambiguous research proposals unethical.

He called this "prevalence-induced concept change." Essentially "problem creep." It explains that as we experience fewer problems, we don't become more satisfied. We just lower our threshold for what we consider a problem. We end up with the same number of troubles. Except our new problems are progressively more hollow.

So Levari got to the heart of why many people can find an issue in nearly any situation, no matter how good we can have it relative to the grand sweep of humanity. We are always moving the goalpost. There is, quite literally, a scientific basis for first-world problems.

"[I] think this is a low-level feature of human psychology," Levari said. The human brain likely evolved to make these relative comparisons, because doing so uses far less brainpower than remembering every instance of a situation you've seen or been in. This brain mechanism in early humans allowed us to make quick decisions and safely navigate our environments. But applied to today's world? "As people make all these relative judgments," Levari said, "they become less and less satisfied than they used to be with the same thing."

This creep phenomenon applies directly to how we now relate to comfort, said Levari. Call it comfort creep. When a new comfort is introduced, we adapt to it and our old comforts become unacceptable. Today's comfort is tomorrow's discomfort. This leads to a new level of what's considered comfortable.

Stairs were once a new marvel of efficiency. But why take them after the advent of the escalator? A little hard-earned lean meat and some plain potatoes was once the best meal of the year. But why have that bland combo when there are restaurants on every block offering perfectly formulated combinations of sugar, salt, and fat? A chilly teepee, yurt, or simple cabin was once a luxurious respite from the weather. But now we can dial our indoor temperatures to our exact specifications.

What's more, new comforts have moved the goalpost further away from what we consider an acceptable level of discomfort. Each advancement shrinks our comfort zones. The critical point, Levari told me, is that this all occurs unconsciously. We are terrible at noticing that comfort creep is consuming us, and what it's doing to us.

So what would happen if we could dissolve our surrounding shades of gray and become aware of comfort creep?

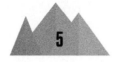

20 YARDS

I FIRST MET Donnie in the fall of 2017.

I'd been commissioned by a national magazine to write about profound changes in the hunting world. There is a growing group of men and women who are squashing the stereotype of hunters being only doughy, bucktoothed Bubbas. They're the opposite of the hunters who drive to the edge of the civilized world and sit around snacking as they wait for some naive, majestic animal to saunter out into a clearing so they can shoot it from afar and add a new decoration to their office wall. That's not the type of hunting our forefathers did. It's not the type of hunting Donnie does, either.

He's a de facto leader of a small but swelling tribe of backcountry hunters. These people are equal parts hunter, ultra-endurance athlete, locavore, survivalist, and naturalist. Donnie has spent half his life living something like our ancestors. He escapes for months at a time into the world's most beautiful, remote, and harsh landscapes while carrying on his back everything he needs to survive. A successful hunt means he'll have to pack out the animal in 70- to 100-pound sections across rugged miles to a pickup location. His biggest haul? Fourteen trips, 100 pounds each of Yukon moose. He utilizes every usable ounce of the animal, providing his family and friends with meat that offers all the Whole Foods upsells: antibiotic- and pesticide-free, grass-fed, and free range to the extreme.

First light was meeting the neon of The Strip as I left the city limits of Las Vegas and turned onto US 93, a two-lane highway that cuts north-south across Nevada's Great Basin. I drove four hours through desert where the jackrabbits outnumbered the passing cars and even the AM dial was useless. I wound up in Ely, Nevada, a town whose elevation number is bigger than its population.

Donnie jumped out of an F-250 pickup and strode toward me. He was wearing a flannel shirt and oversize boots. His shoulder-length gray hair flowed out from under a Filson watch cap. Picture a bearded, frontier Fabio.

He reached out a rough hand to shake mine and went full-on Ranger Rick. "I've been up there for a week now, and, man, it's beautiful. This is fantastic, fantastic country," he said. Then he inhaled the sagey Nevada air and looked toward the 10,000-foot peaks of the White Pine Mountains. "Let's head up."

Donnie piloted the Ford down an empty highway. He eventually turned onto a bumpy, sagebrush-flanked dirt back road. We passed a pulled-over pickup surrounded by a group of generously bellied, camouflaged men using binoculars to scope the mountain ranges above. "Many guys here stay in a local hotel and hunt from the road," said Donnie, shaking his head.

He turned the truck out of the high desert and onto a rocky 4x4 road leading into a dark canyon. Donnie began admitting to me that he gets more out of the spiritual, physical process of stalking prey for weeks on end across fantastic places than he does from the kill itself. The process is the reward. But a successful outcome makes the process that much more rewarding.

"I didn't come from a hunting and fishing family," he said. "As a kid I got an *Outdoor Life* book subscription and became obsessed. I wanted those big adventures. During my freshman year of college I headed up to Prince William Sound for a black bear hunt."

We awkwardly bounced up the rough road, leaning into each of the big ruts the truck crawled over. "I was obsessed about getting a bear and packing it out," he said. "I'd made my way over to this remote beach on Whale Bay when the first bear walked up. I completely forgot what I was there for. I watched how his feet hit the rocks, how he'd pick up salmon and eat it. I noticed all of the super-intricate details of his face and eyes and how he breathed. I was blown away. So connected to that bear. I got a really heavy heart and almost started to tear up."

The road terminated at a trailhead deep inside the piney canyon. We hopped out of the truck's cab and Donnie began stuffing gear into his pack. No camo. Instead, dark technical outdoor gear you'd find at REI instead of Cabela's. Adventure gear like ultralight down mid-layers and GORE-TEX shells designed for mountaineers, he said, fit and perform better. They also make him more approachable to nonhunters. "Most big game can only see in grayscale, anyways," he said. "Big game camo is mostly a marketing ploy."

He continued the story. "I just couldn't shoot that bear. Later that night the captain of the boat I was staying on told me, 'I think you're a hunter. I think you'll be disappointed if you don't leave here with a bear,'" said Donnie. We were trudging the steep, pine-flanked trail as the canyon became darker with the falling sun.

"The next day I went back to the beach. It was surrounded by snowcapped peaks, and it was just unbelievably beautiful. There were bald eagles hunting fish. The bay was blood red from a killer whale hunting a humpback whale calf. And then a bear came out of the forest. I aimed and paused," he said as we passed a rocky creek. "Then I shot. The bear hit the ground. And then it all hit me really heavy. The bear wasn't going to go on being a bear anymore. And that was on me. But after sitting awhile I noticed the eagles and whales again.

They were all hunting. There were ravens flying overhead waiting to pick the remains of their kills and my bear. It was like, 'Oh, OK, I've inserted myself into this ecosystem. I'm just another part of this natural process.'"

He's been part of the process ever since. After college, Donnie signed on to be a field biologist for the US Fish and Wildlife Service. He'd spend six months at a time surveying salmon counts on Alaska's Tuluksak River. "I was alone up there. I lived out of a three-man yellow tent," he said. "I'd see another human every three weeks, when my supervisor would come to drop off supplies. I'd fish for my dinner alongside a pack of wolves."

He eventually began filming his adventures. Partly to add evidence to his Jack London–esque stories, and partly to show people what they're missing. He first shot with a cheap handheld camera. Then he met William, who'd been filming his own hunts in the Northeast. They created a hunting documentary, which they called *The River's Divide.* It's nothing like the stuff you might see on the Outdoors Channel. "So many hunting films and shows celebrate death. 'Whack 'em and stack 'em,' they say. It's gross, just gross," said Donnie. His films are more like *Planet Earth,* but with hunting. Long, quiet shots of, say, a misty fall morning at a pond, or extended footage of a fox who wandered into camp.

The River's Divide covers Donnie's four-year odyssey searching for a Badlands whitetail he named Steve. It focuses on the buck's habitat, evolution, and personality, along with the conflicted emotions Donnie felt after the kill. "I got thousands of letters from hunters and nonhunters alike after that. People liked my approach. They also connected with the movies, I think, because they show the value of breaking out of the modern rat race and being present in and a part of nature."

Donnie now spends months each year out of the rat race, exploring hundreds of miles of untamed, remote regions of the Arctic, Mexico, Russia, Alaska, the Yukon, and more. "If you want to have amazing experiences," he said as we wove up the trail, the silhouette of towering pines black against the moonlit navy sky, "you have to put yourself in amazing places." The guy is a far-out mix of Davy Crockett, David Attenborough, and the Dalai Lama.

When we arrived at our first camping spot, it was a kind of dark I'd never encounter in Las Vegas. A patch of rocky ground was the only semi-flat space we could find in a pitchy mountain meadow. I filled my water bottle at a spring seeping from the hillside and took a long drink. I was shaking.

It was nearly freezing outside. Apparently my 72-degree lifestyle—going from temperature-controlled home to car, to office, to home—hadn't exactly readied my brain and body for any type of weather that was not . . . 72 degrees. I was feeling the kind of cold that travels up your extremities and into the center of your core. So I put on every single layer I'd packed. A wool T-shirt, a wool midweight layer, a down vest, a jacket, hat, and gloves. I still shivered like a fool.

William stood stoically near the spring wearing a short-sleeve T-shirt, stone dead to the temperature. "Aren't you cold?" I asked.

"Huh?" he said, apparently unaware of the frost exiting his mouth in the reply. "Cold," I said, pulling on the sleeve of my jacket. "Aren't you cold?"

"Oh, no. Not really. I get that it's cold out," said William. "But it doesn't bother me. I kind of like how it feels. I can usually wear a T-shirt down to forty degrees."

We all convened to eat dinner in Donnie's four-man teepee (which sounds weird, but it's basically just a tent with a higher roof and no floor cover). I wasn't antihunting. But I also wasn't ready to pick up a gun or bow. So I asked Donnie, Why hunt at all? Trophy hunting to me seems abhorrent. Meat is readily available in every restaurant and grocery store.

He agreed with me about trophy hunting. Then he explained to me the strict ethical code that he'd developed during his work as a wildlife biology researcher. For example, he only hunts older

members of a species, because removing an old animal often improves the health of the herd as a whole, while taking a young animal
does the opposite. It also allows youngsters to live out a full life. He
adds that he's sometimes, much to his annoyance, confused with a
trophy hunter. "I'm definitely not chasing antlers or horns," he said.
"But older animals often have the largest antlers and horns."

Donnie sat back onto his sleeping pad to get philosophical. "We
came up through an ecosystem of predator and prey. If you asked a
rabbit, 'Why are you a rabbit?' he'd probably say, 'I don't know. I'm
just a rabbit. I eat carrots and I have this poufy tail and floppy ears.
I've always been a rabbit.' So that's kind of my answer, too," Donnie
said. "I'm a hunter. When you peel back all the layers, I think humans basically evolved from single-celled organisms, into apes, into
humans. We are animals. And we are fundamentally hunting and
gathering animals. Most of us still partake in some level of predator-
prey relationship. Hunting and gathering. Because most of us still
eat meat, and all of us still eat vegetables," he said. "But we now have
the luxury of having all of our hunting and gathering done for us at
an industrial scale. If we didn't have that, I guarantee we'd all still be
doing our own hunting and gathering. I think I'm just closer to our
original form compared to most people."

Then he paused for a time. "Look, I know hunting is controver-
sial," he said. "But if you eat meat, your barrier to entry is likely going
into the grocery and swiping a credit card. You don't know anything
about the animal. How it lived, where it came from, or what kind of
life it had. Well, I know."

We talked a lot about meat during dinner. But there wasn't much
to the actual meal. Just some reconstituted backpacking mush. Afterward I retreated to my modest quarters—a tarp propped up by a
trekking pole—and tried to get some sleep.

The trip would only get more uncomfortable from there. Over
the next few days we would climb steep, untamed hills for hours on
end with 60-pound packs on our backs. Getting water in the high

country required descending thousands of feet to a spring below and then toting the heavy, awkward water bags back up to camp. When we weren't hiking, we were sitting atop windswept peaks, using a spotting scope to look for elk. Except we had just one spotting scope and I had no clue where to look. So I sat in a state of boredom I hadn't experienced since I was a junior high student waiting for algebra class to end. To keep our packs lighter we subsisted on a Snickers bar or two and a freeze-dried meal each day. That's enough food for an Instagram model, maybe. But it surely wasn't enough for a grown man who'd spent all day huffing a heavy pack uphill. I was ravenous. I also didn't shower or wash my hands the entire time, an oddity in the age of Purell. Nor did I remove my layers, gloves, or hat.

I spent a lot of time questioning the necessity of the whole endeavor.

But after a few days of hiking the 10,000-foot granite and limestone ridges among bristlecones—2,000-year-old pines that exist only in the West's harshest, highest landscapes—we experienced a close encounter.

"Get down," Donnie whisper-shouted.

A pickup-truck-size bull elk stood 60 yards ahead. His rear end faced us as he bowed down his neck to eat grass, his antlers sweeping the dry mountain air like construction cranes. We hit the dirt. If the elk smelled us, he'd break into a 40-mile-an-hour gallop, out of sight and range.

Donnie nocked an arrow in his bow and began an exaggerated, cartoonish tiptoe toward the elk. At 20 yards out, we crouched behind a granite boulder and waited. We were looking for the animal to show us his shoulder. The arrow would hopefully silently and cleanly enter there, slicing its way across the dorsal aorta and into the lung. A couple of seconds of life, at most, after a shot like that. Arrows are silent and sharp. The animal often topples over before becoming aware of its deathly predicament.

The bull stopped chewing. His dark eyes seemed to squint as his white-and-brown ears drew back. He lifted his head and turned to inspect his surroundings. This exposed his vital area. Donnie pulled his bow to full draw.

Zen monks meditate for decades to achieve the state of presence I discovered. My senses converged on that elk and my relation to it. I was aware of the thick texture of its fur and the way it elegantly transitioned from tan to brown to white. I noticed the knobs, shallow curves, and sharp points of its overbuilt antlers. I heard its teeth masticating the grass, his heavy breaths picking up and swelling his rib cage.

I had never been so close to death, the moment where the life cycle ends for one living thing so that it may continue for another. The last meat I'd eaten came in a paper bag and between a bun, and was likely shipped from some secretive midwestern slaughterhouse.

I wondered only if Donnie was going to let that arrow fly, 200 miles an hour into that unassuming bull. Until I became aware of a spectator. A coyote lurked behind us, anticipating a dinner of elk entrails. The elk became aware, too, and he spooked, galloping off as Donnie muscled the bow string back to a rest. "He was big and beautiful, but he was too young," Donnie said.

Smoke from western wildfires was filtering the sun a maroon shade as we walked the ridges back to camp. I felt more alive than I had since my early days of sobriety, when I realized I had a whole new life ahead of me. My mind was quieter, my body abler. I felt more in tune with higher rhythms than with the frenetic frequencies of modern life.

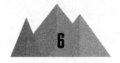

50/50

WHEN I RETURNED to "civilization," the discomfort-induced buzz hung around for weeks. I kept returning in my head to how I felt during those wild days, ascending unforgiving mountain faces, missing meals, attempting in vain to escape the cold, never knowing what the untamed world would throw at me next. It was feeling the opposite of comfort creep. It was, I'd soon learn from a Harvard-educated doctor, a type of *misogi*.

The *Kojiki* is a Japanese document commissioned by Empress Genmei in the year AD 711. It's the oldest living document in Japan. It includes myths, legends, and historical accounts of the Japanese archipelago, the formation of heaven and earth, and the origins of Shinto gods and heroes. The *Kojiki*'s most epic tale spawned misogi.

Izanagi was a god in the Shinto faith and was married to the Shinto goddess of creation and death. Things were perfect for the two gods, until Izanagi's wife died in childbirth. She descended into the Land of the Dead, the underworld where all Shinto gods go in the afterlife.

The Shinto god was wrecked. He wept and slumbered through life until he decided he just couldn't live that way anymore. He made up his mind to venture into the Land of the Dead to bring back his wife.

Izanagi entered a cavern that led into the underworld. As he journeyed deeper he encountered a hellish landscape. There were demons, zombies, and grotesque figures who wanted to capture him and keep him there for eternity.

Despite all of hell working to stop him, Izanagi pushed on and found his wife. But he was terrified to see that she'd succumbed to hell's perils. She was partially decomposed and demonic-looking. He realized he'd be next to fall to the underworld's defilements if he didn't escape quickly.

So Izanagi made a fantastic break through the caverns of hell. Demons and monsters grabbed at him, trying to pull him downward. Failure seemed imminent. He nearly gave up. But he dug deep mentally and physically, kept pushing, and eventually burst from the cavern's entrance.

Izanagi then dove into a nearby freezing river to purify himself from the degradations of hell. The experience rocketed him into a state of *sumikiri,* pure clarity of mind and body, and removed all his impurities, weaknesses, and past limits. It made him tougher in mind, body, and spirit.

The state of sumikiri provided by misogi is why ancient students of aikido would immerse themselves in natural bodies of cold water. Waterfalls, streams, or the ocean would wash away their defilements and reconnect them with the universe. More recently, the idea of misogi has been applied to other forms of using epic challenges in nature to cleanse the defilements of the modern world. These modern misogis offer a hard brain, body, and spirit reboot. They help their practitioners smash previous limits and deliver the mindful, centering confidence and competence the Japanese aikido followers were also seeking. Dr. Marcus Elliott pioneered this new brand of misogi. And he's convinced it works.

When I contacted Elliott about misogi, he first let me know that he was tired of talking numbers and figures about NBA players and the biomechanics of twisted ankles, compressive loads of a vertical jump, and eccentric forces applied during the step-back three-pointer. "I assumed you were reaching out about athlete data and modeling.

Which I love," said Elliott, a Harvard-trained physician who owns P3, a sports science facility that uses deep biometric data to improve pro athlete performance. "But I don't really want to talk about that."

The *Wall Street Journal* had just visited Elliott's Santa Barbara–based facility, an unmarked warehouse gym filled with fitness equipment, computers, and scientific gizmos. The newspaper was profiling Elliott and his work with Luka Doncic, the 2018 NBA Rookie of the Year, All-Star, etc.

At just 15 years old, Doncic began traveling the 6,000 miles from his home in Slovenia to P3. There Elliott discovered the secret sauce of Luka's game. Elliott and his team of PhDs attached reflective markers all over the kid—his torso, back, legs, knees, ankles, feet, and more. Then Doncic went through all the motions he might use in a game. Meanwhile, a movie set's worth of 3D cameras rolled and captured more than 5,000 data points. With that information, Elliott could see the movement asymmetries that might be setting Doncic up for injury, and what physical skills he was good and bad at.

The data showed Doncic couldn't jump to save his life. But he was incredibly gifted at applying "eccentric force." This basically means that Luka is fast at slowing down. Elliott's advice: Luka should develop his game around plays where he sprints forward, stops abruptly, and shoots, leaving his defender still careening forward as the shot arcs toward the hoop.

Luka did just that. Now the kid's the future of the NBA. Roughly 60 percent of NBA players have come through P3 to uncover the perils and opportunities hidden within their movement patterns.

Fascinating stuff. But it's not what I wanted to talk about either. I had misogi on my mind, and that's what Elliott wanted to hear. "If we can really dig into misogi," he said, "I'm game to having you come down."

And so it was, a handful of months later, that I found myself hammering up a cliffside trail above Santa Barbara with Elliott. We'd powered through creeks and over boulders. We'd zoomed through rock gardens and abundantly green forests that smelled like fresh eucalyptus. After we bounded up a punishingly steep section with a view of the ocean, we both doubled over, hands to knees, to suck air.

"Over our species' hundreds of thousands of years of evolution," Elliott said, "it was essential for our survival to do hard shit all the time. To be challenged. And this was without safety nets. These challenges could be from hunts, getting resources for the tribe, moving from summering to wintering grounds, and so on. Each time we took on one of these challenges we'd learn what our potential is."

Elliott is six foot one with the trim 190-pound build of a triathlete. Picture a younger, tanner, SoCal cross between Dennis Quaid and Bruce Springsteen. He's 54, but I would have believed him had he told me he was 40.

"In modern society, however," Elliott said, "it's suddenly possible to survive without being challenged. You'll still have plenty of food. You'll have a comfortable home. A good job to show up to, and some people who love you. And that seems like an OK life, right?

"But," he said, sweeping his arm to create a big imaginary circle that encompassed the trail and foliage flanking it. "Let's say your potential is this big circle."

Then he pulled his hands into his chest and made a dinner-plate-size circle in the exact middle of the much larger circle. "Well, most of us live in this small space right here. We have no idea what exists on the edges of our potential. And by not having any idea what it's like out on the edge . . . man, we really miss something vital."

A salty wind was blowing over the ocean and sidling up into the hills. It passed over my sweat-soaked T-shirt as Elliott continued. "I believe people have innate evolutionary machinery that gets triggered when they go out and do really fucking hard things. When they explore those edges of their comfort zone."

Enter misogi, a circumnavigation of the edges of human potential.

Each year for the last quarter century Elliott has undertaken one of these epic, far-out challenges. "Think of it this way," he said. "In the gym, I identify a problem an athlete has that is putting him or her at risk. Then I use the artificial construct of the gym environment to improve that athlete's performance when he or she goes into the unpredictable, unstructured Wild West of a game."

A hiker with a black Lab passed us on her way down. Elliott and I both patted the dog.

"Misogis are that same concept. Except for the modern condition. In misogi we're using the artificial, contrived concept of going out and doing a hard task to mimic these challenges that humans used to face all the time. These challenges that our environment used to naturally show us that we're so removed from now," he said. "Then when we return to the Wild West of our everyday lives we are better for it. We have the right tools for the job."

The practice has cranked the dial of his physical, mental, and spiritual health and potential, he said. And done the same for the other seekers who've joined him.

There is, for example, Nelson Parrish, a 40-something Santa Barbara artist whose work melds painting, sculpted metals, and natural woods. The work is "contextualized through the verbiage of speed and language of color," Parrish told me. Its goal is to force the viewer to "disengage from the peripheral" and force a consideration of "the expansion and contraction of time." The work's been featured in *Vogue* magazine and is collected by the Hermès family, Rob Lowe, John Legend, and more.

"Misogi is not about physical accomplishment," said Parrish. "It asks, 'What are you mentally and spiritually willing to put yourself through to be a better human?' Misogis have allowed me to let go of fear and anxiousness, and you can see that in my work."

There is also Kyle Korver, the NBA All-Star and jump-shot artist who is fourth on the all-time three-pointer list. Korver credits his most clutch performances to the lessons of misogi.

"One year we carried an eighty-five-pound rock five kilometers underwater," said Elliott, speaking of a misogi Parrish and Korver participated in. That misogi occurred just a few miles downhill from this trail, along the coast of Santa Barbara Island. One guy would dive anywhere from seven to ten feet down. He'd pick up the rock and cradle it, then walk the ocean floor as far as he could (maybe 10 to 20 yards). Then another guy would dive down and do the same. And so on and so forth until after five hours the rock was at point B.

"Another year we stand-up paddleboarded twenty-five miles across the Santa Barbara Channel," said Elliott. "We'd only paddleboarded a few times before that. Waves kept knocking us into the ocean every ten minutes. We couldn't think about crossing the full channel. Instead we had to focus on the process in front of us. Keeping our balance and getting in one perfect stroke. Then one more perfect stroke. And eventually we looked up and were across an ocean."

Korver said the paddleboard misogi led him to break the NBA record for the most consecutive games with a three-pointer. As he inched toward the record, his teammates would remind him that he had only, say, 12 more games with a three-pointer to go. He'd tell them that all he cared about was the next perfect stroke.

Misogi may uncover the coveted "flow state."

As a young psychology researcher in the 1960s, Mihaly Csikszentmihalyi noticed something fascinating about artists. They could become completely present and engrossed in their work. In these instances their action and awareness would merge. Random thoughts, bodily sensations like pain or hunger, and even their sense of ego and self would all fade. It was a sort of prolonged Zen in the art of . . . art.

So he began studying the state, which he eventually named "flow state." Over Csikszentmihalyi's career—where he ran the psychology department at the University of Chicago and was president of the American Psychology Association—he interviewed thousands of high-level performers. They ranged from chess players, rock climbers, and painters to surgeons, writers, and Formula 1 drivers.

Lapsing into flow requires two conditions: The task must stretch a person's limits and it must have a clear goal. The flow state, Csik-szentmihalyi and the other researchers now believe, is a key driver of happiness and growth. It is the opposite of apathy. Csikszentmihalyi wrote that flow has the "potential to make life more rich, intense, and meaningful; it is good because it increases the strengths and complexity of the self."

ELLIOTT GREW UP PLAYING ANY SPORT HE COULD—FOOTBALL, BASEBALL, ETC.—AND developed an early obsession with physiology and human performance. The interest ran so deep that in his teens he asked his parents for a subscription to the academic journal *Medicine & Science in Sports & Exercise* for Christmas.

Elliott planned to play college ball but injured himself in high school. He jumped around universities. Transferred from UC Berkeley to UC Santa Barbara to Harvard.

"After I recovered from the injury, I still needed some way to physically challenge myself. So I got into endurance sports," he said. "In college I didn't ever party. All I did was train and study like a madman. I lived out of a VW van for a few years. It all was very simple. I had just a few belongings. If I ended the day fitter or smarter, then it was a good day."

Elliott won some big races, landed a sponsorship with Nike, and made the top ten in world triathlete rankings. He applied to Harvard Medical School and an MIT PhD program in biomechanics, the study of biological systems through mechanical principles. Both schools offered him a spot.

"I had no desire to be a doctor. But I ended up going to medical school because I thought it would be more interesting," he said. "One moment I'd be cutting someone open and the next dealing with a psych patient."

He quit triathlons in medical school. "When I started racing I'd already decided I was going to quit when I was twenty-five," he said. Needing to spend 100 hours a week in class, on rounds, and studying didn't help, either.

But all of that silent, solitary time running, riding, or swimming—becoming comfortable with discomfort, persisting despite all of his biological impulses telling him to slow down or tap out—had remodeled his psyche. "Endurance sports gave me some understanding of what it was to push to deeper levels and find new layers within myself," he told me. "When I stopped doing triathlons, I still had this sense of adventure. This need to explore those edges where I'd find a new, better part of myself."

So Elliot began doing what he initially called "these kooky challenges." Once or twice a year he'd take on an unstructured difficult task. For instance, "After finishing rounds I drove all night to [New Hampshire's] White Mountains, sleep deprived and running on hospital food, and decided to hike to the top of the farthest peak in one day, with no preparation," he said. "It was all just to see if I could. I'd get to what I thought was my edge, but I'd keep going. Then eventually I'd realize I was way past my old edge and still going. And so that edge was now in a different place than when I started. And that was so satisfying, so satisfying."

One year Elliott and a med school friend, Garth Meckler, flew into Riverton, Wyoming, for one of the "kooky adventures."

"We hitched a ride on a post office truck from the airport out to a trailhead. And then we powered out a fifteen-hour day into the wilderness with eighty-pound packs on our back. We were just kicking each other's asses," Elliott said. "Garth was an Olympic-level judo competitor. And as we were hiking he told me about this thing that his judo dojo borrowed from the samurai, who borrowed it from aikido, who borrowed it from these ancient Japanese religious texts. And it was called a misogi challenge. So I started calling these kooky challenges 'misogi,' as a tip of the hat to Garth and as a recognition that trying really hard shit is purifying and life enhancing."

Elliott graduated from medical school $330,000 in debt. "My instructors at Harvard wanted me to be an academic. But I just wasn't built to be caged in a lab, hospital, or office. I wanted to be on the ground and really affect things," he said.

Team athletic training at the time hadn't evolved much past tweaking sets and reps. "It was really clear in my mind that there was going to be value in applying more science to sport, and that if I didn't try it I'd always regret it," said Elliott. "But I needed a real problem to solve."

The New England Patriots had a problem. They were at the time a mediocre football team racked with an average of 21.5 hamstring injuries a year. Elliott took a scientist's approach to the issue. He studied years of player data on the injury's common origins and tested the team. Then he took a physician's approach to the solution. He developed individualized player training prescriptions that he believed would reduce the chance of the injury, even though he'd been told by his instructors that "exercise medicine was a waste of a world-class education."

His work dropped the Patriots' hamstring injury rate to just three a season. "Won a couple Super Bowls with the team," said Elliott.

Next he became the MLB's first Director of Sports Science and Performance. And now he's "doing this basketball thing." P3 opened in 2006. Elliott is considered a pioneer and one of the world's foremost sports scientists. His brand is officially partnered with the NBA, and his client list is a who's who of the game: James Harden, Kawhi Leonard, Giannis Antetokounmpo, Doncic, and many more. He's also continued working with individual pros in sports across the board and is beginning to consult for world soccer and NASCAR.

Recently, Harvard Medical School awarded Elliott with one of its highest honors, the Augustus Thorndike Visiting Lecturer Award. "It's funny that the same people who were telling me I was wasting my time said 'Come back and teach us,'" said Elliott.

The misogis have continued—one a year—and Elliott credits them with his ability to affect things in his personal and professional life.

"Misogis can show you that you had this latent potential you didn't realize, and that you can go further than you ever believed. When you put yourself in a challenging environment where you have a good chance of failing, lots of fears fade and things start moving."

ELLIOTT STEPPED FORWARD TO GIVE ME A POUND, THEN TURNED AND BOUNDED DOWN the trail, his chiseled legs a pair of pistons kicking up dust. We eventually ascended into a shady forest, where the trail flattened.

"In our model of misogi, there are only two rules," said Elliott. "Rule number one is that it has to be really fucking hard. Rule number two is that you can't die."

I understood the not-dying part, but asked him how he determines if something is hard enough.

"We're generally guided by the idea that you should have a fifty percent chance of success—*if you do everything right*," he said. "So if you decided you wanted to run a twenty-five-mile trail, and you're preparing by working up to a twenty-mile training run and doing thirty-five or forty miles a week of running . . . that's not a misogi. Your chance of failure is too low. But if you've never run more than ten miles, think you could probably run fifteen, but are iffy on whether you could run twenty . . . then that twenty-five miles is probably a misogi."

This rule also renders misogi a moving target. One person's 50 percent is often not the same as another's. "If someone has never run more than a couple miles, then a 10K could be a misogi," said Elliott. Modern humans may have an unmet need to do what's truly difficult for us. New research shows that depression, anxiety, and feeling like you don't belong can be linked to being untested.

"So you must fail about half the time?" I asked.

"I've actually failed my last couple misogis," he said.

Elliott's most recent was a rim-to-rim-to-rim run of the Grand Canyon. A 46-mile physical moonshot with roughly 22,000 feet of elevation change.

"I hadn't run for years," he said. "But I put in a couple of eighteen-mile runs beforehand."

He failed. Hard. "I really blew up my knees on the descent off the South Rim," he said. "Once we made it up to the North Rim we began descending back down to the canyon floor. I realized I wasn't going to make it. If I continued I'd probably have to be helicoptered out of there. So I hiked back up to the North Rim and managed to chase down the last four-hour shuttle back to the South Rim, where I'd parked."

The forest opened into a steep section. "And I can tell you," he said through heavy breaths as we powered up a hill, "the human brain hates this construct. The brain wants nothing to do with failure. *Especially* if you execute perfectly on your side."

It's a hardwired phenomenon. Scientists at the University of Michigan investigated the evolutionary origins of fear. They say our current fears are often driven by our past lifestyles. Early humans used to regularly face potentially lethal danger from hungry predators and venomous snakes, members of other tribes, violent weather and treacherous landscapes, loss of social status, and so on.*

This is why humans today can still easily spot rustling in bushes or snakes slithering through the grass. Why we're wary of strangers. Why we avoid bad weather and heights. Why we become anxious when we have to stick our necks out in public, like with public speaking.

"Failure even a hundred years ago could mean that you die," said Elliott. "But people *vastly* overestimate the consequences of failure today. Failure now is that you fuck up a PowerPoint presentation and your boss gives you a bad look."

The human mind is programmed to overestimate the consequences of something like screwing up a PowerPoint, because past social

---

* This also explains why humans have undersize fears of some of the modern ways we die. Like car accidents.

failures often got us kicked out of the tribe, after which we'd usually die at the hands of nature, according to those Michigan scientists.

"So this evolutionary machinery we have doesn't serve us anymore," Elliott said. "Because I can tell you that nothing great in life comes with complete assurance of success. Engaging in an environment where there's a high probability of failure, even if you execute perfectly, has huge ramifications for helping you lose a fear of failing. Huge ramifications for showing you what your potential is.

"Looking back on the rim-to-rim-to-rim run . . . ," he said through exasperated breaths, "I hadn't even run twenty miles. My chance of making it wasn't even close to fifty percent. Not even close. It was so far from fifty. It was probably ten or fifteen. But standing on the edge of the South Rim of the Grand Canyon at the beginning . . . even if I didn't feel superhuman, I felt like I had the right tools to go explore this thing. Powers beyond what was obvious to me. There's adventure in that."

Variations of the misogi myth exist through time and space. Greek, Mesopotamian, Buddhist, Norse, Christian, Hindu, and ancient Egyptian mythology all have some version of what Joseph Campbell called "the hero's journey." The hero exits the comfort of home for adventure. He's hit with a challenge. It tests his physical, psychological, and spiritual fortitude. He struggles. Yet he manages to prevail. He returns with heightened knowledge, skills, confidence, and experience, and a clearer sense of his or her place in the world. And research going back to the late 1800s proves that mere mortals benefit from epic physical trials.

ARNOLD VAN GENNEP, BORN IN 1873, WAS BRILLIANT BUT ALWAYS A PROPER PAIN IN the ass. His teachers in his French elementary school reported that van Gennep was smart but a "terrible boy," so his parents dumped him into boarding school. There he kept up his reputation. The kid was a valedictorian who had a standing meeting in the principal's office.

Van Gennep's stepfather, a surgeon, wanted him to follow in the old man's footsteps and study surgery, in Lyon. Van Gennep decided he'd rather study the topic in Paris. The stepfather wouldn't concede. So van Gennep decided he'd irk the old man a step further. He wouldn't go into medicine at all. Instead he'd study languages and anthropology. Van Gennep could, by his own admission, speak "18 languages and a fair amount of dialects." That talent sparked in him an interest in other cultures.

After college van Gennep began translating anthropological studies. Thanks to colonialism, studies were rushing in from many different countries, all in different languages. Van Gennep became a terminal for this new research. He translated fieldwork about people who lived around the world, in places ranging from the plains of Mongolia and North America to the islands of Fiji and Greece. He quickly discovered a unique commonality among these far-off bands of humans. Men and women in these cultures undertook a physical, nature-based rite of passage.

For example, the young men of the Aboriginal people, Australian natives who have lived on the island continent for some 65,000 years, went on "walkabout." They'd venture alone for up to six months into the Australian outback, a place that's essentially uninhabitable. Its temperatures can reach above 100 degrees Fahrenheit in the summer. Its venomous snakes are among the deadliest in the world. The person was toast if he hadn't prepared for the quest by practicing skills like building a shelter, hunting and foraging for food, learning which plants act as medicine, and anything else that he might need in order not to die. Or he'd come back into camp a failure, if he came back at all.

But if the person made it, he'd return to the tribe physically and mentally tougher and more capable, with a greater understanding of the world and his place in it.

The Inuit have a similar tradition. It's not quite as long or lonely, but it's a lot colder. When Inuit children appear strong enough, usually around age 12, elders lead them out into the Arctic for their first hunt. They bring tents, spears, and other necessities, and eat what they kill. The journey takes place across miles and weeks, and the young person must down a narwhal, caribou, or bearded seal. The kids pick up valuable survival skills and evolve as people. The journey also hammers them with the harsh weather of the Arctic. This toughens them while also teaching them skills they need to thrive.

Then there's the rite of passage of the Maasai, a tribe who lives in Kenya and Tanzania. Young Maasai men were sent alone into the savanna to hunt a male lion. Not with a rifle or a bow. With a spear.

These solo lion hunts required an unbelievable amount of training. A person needed strength, endurance, undaunted courage, and hunting skills that he'd literally bet his life on. These men didn't sneak up on a sleeping lion. They'd chase it while rattling bells at it, to compel the lion to square off with the skinny hunters face-to-face.

If the Maasai man succeeded, he'd have completed the ultimate physical and mental challenge and officially transitioned into a warrior. Or he failed and officially transitioned into dinner for a pride of lions. As the Maasai Association, a group that preserves and celebrates Maasai heritage, casually notes, "Many warriors have been lost to lions."

The Nez Perce, Native Americans who live in the Pacific Northwest, went on vision quests. They'd walk into the mountains or desert unarmed and without food to spend about a week in solitude. They'd fast and drink little water, expose themselves to the elements, and go without shelter or fire. Yellow Wolf, a Nez Perce warrior who fought in the Nez Perce War of 1877, explained that the process developed "strength to help you in dangers, in battle." These types of mind-body-and-spirit-strengthening vision quests were common among many indigenous American tribes.

"The idea of a rite of passage is that the elders are seeing in you the potential to rise up and achieve this really important, challenging thing that is going to benefit you and everyone around you on many levels," said Elliott. "They're saying, 'We think you're ready, but you're really going to have to dig deep and find your shit.'"

In 1909 van Gennep wrote a seminal text about these events, which he called *The Rites of Passage*. (He's the person who coined the term.)

He found that these processes—whether walking around the outback, hunting a lion in Kenya, tripping out on the Columbia River Plateau, or perhaps, even, undergoing a misogi—all have three key elements.

The first is separation. The person exits the society in which they live and ventures into the wild. The second is transition. The person enters a challenging middle ground, where they battle with nature and their mind telling them to quit. The third is incorporation. The person completes the challenge and reenters their normal life an improved person. It's an exploration and expansion of the edge of a person's comfort zone.

Misogi, Elliott said, is the same. "Misogis are an emotional, spiritual, and psychological challenge that masquerades as a physical challenge."

As we run, Elliott and I talk about how rites of passage, in the traditional sense, are largely gone. "What do we have now?" he asked.

Rites of passage still exist in a few cultures. The Dutch continue to uphold a scouting tradition called "dropping." It involves blindfolding kids and then dropping them in the woods at night with limited resources to see if they can find their way home. But I don't know anyone whose parents dumped them in the wilderness and said, "See you in six months." Or handed them a crude weapon and said, "Bring me the corpse of the most deadly animal you can find." Society has, in fact, taken an extremely opposite approach.

Scientists at New York University identify 1990 as the beginning of helicopter parenting. The researchers say that's when many parents stopped allowing their children to go outside unsupervised until they were as old as 16, due to unfounded, media-driven fears of kidnapping. We've now deteriorated from helicopter parenting to snowplow parenting. These parents violently force any and all obstacles out of their child's path. Preventing kids from exploring their edges is largely thought to be the cause of the abnormally high and growing rates of anxiety and depression in young people. A study found that anxiety and depression rates in college students rose roughly 80 percent in the generation just after helicopter parenting began. Some states have even had to pass "free-range parenting" laws after some parents were being charged with neglect for letting their kids go outside alone.

I'm old enough that I spent the majority of my youth outside alone or with friends. But as Elliott and I run, I try to think of my own rite of passage. I did attain the Eagle Scout ranking. But even scouting's most challenging outdoor adventures were no-fail propositions. My troop's closest thing to the Dutch practice of dropping was the Wilderness Survival merit badge exercise. But the test was constantly being canceled due to bad weather, ironically.

Anthony Stevens, a Jungian psychologist, has spent a career studying archetypes and rites of passage. He believes these rites are fundamental to the human experience, a sort of crossing of a line in the sand that makes humans *human*.

"Although our culture has allowed (rites of passage) to atrophy with disuse," he wrote, "there persists in all of us an archetypal need to be initiated."

IT WAS 7:35 P.M. AND ELLIOTT AND I WERE AT HIS HOME IN THE SANTA BARBARA hills. After our run we hung around the P3 facility. Then we cruised up to his house and had just finished dinner, a lasagna prepared by his wife, Nadine. She was born in a small village in Bavaria and moved across the United States racking up degree after degree until she met Elliott. She's tall and blond and the opposite of a helicopter parent. Nadine encourages her kids to surf and go on mini-misogis with her husband. But she also enforces misogi rule number two, don't die.

"We all have families," said Elliott. "So the worst case of misogi is that you fail. And maybe you had a long day and it might leave a few scars. But you can't die. And that rule is pretty simple."

"How do you"—I searched for the right words to use in front of Nadine—"make sure you don't break rule number two?"

"During a misogi you definitely don't feel like you're in control," said Elliott. "But you won't die. You do have to ensure you'll be safe. We had a safety dive team present in the underwater rock misogi. In the channel crossing we had a safety boat."

Toward the end of the evening, Elliott mentioned to me that he has a couple of softer rules for misogis. He described them as guidelines more than hard rules. One was that the misogi should be "quirky. Creative. Far out. Something uncommon."

"Moving an eighty-five-pound rock five kilometers underwater?" I asked.

He smiled. "Yes. And the reason for this is because the more quirky the misogi, the less chance you can compare it to anything else," he said. "It's important to take on challenges that are *your* challenges. Misogi is you against you. It's against this phenomenon of 'Oh, that guy did this thing in this amount of time and I'm going to try to do it faster.' Because that's comparison shopping. And that's just such a shitty way to go through life."

Parrish talked at length about this guideline. He summed it up like this: "When you remove superficial metrics you can accomplish way more."

Which brought Elliott to guideline two: Don't advertise misogi. It's OK to talk about misogi with friends and family. But you don't Tweet, Instagram, Facebook, or boast about misogi.

"Everyone today has such outward-facing lives," said Elliott. "They do stuff so they can post on social media about some badass thing they did to get a bunch of likes.

"Misogis are inward facing," he said. "A big part of the value proposition is that I'm going to do something that's really uncomfortable. I'm going to want to quit. And it's going to be hard not to quit because no one is watching. But I'm not going to quit because *I'm* watching. And then I can reflect back on how I was the only person watching myself and I still rose to the occasion in a big way. There's some deep satisfaction in that. Did you really do what you think is the right thing when you were the only person watching? Or do you need an audience or a big pat on the back for that? Are you not important enough to do it for you? We had this guideline before social media, and it seems more relevant today."

Elliott is an impressive character, with the Harvard MD and history of improving human performance. But his thrill-seeking "kooky challenges" can sometimes come across as something less than scholarly. After I came out of his charismatic spell I sought out another scientist to learn if there's any science to misogis.

MARK SEERY, PHD, HAS SPENT HIS LIFE STUDYING THE EDGE OF THE HUMAN COMFORT

zone. As a psychologist at the University at Buffalo, Seery was always fascinated by the common cliché "What doesn't kill us makes us stronger." Little quips like that always seem to have a nugget of truth to them. But the data didn't back the saying.

"The existing literature suggested that there was this clear, straightforward relationship where when a bad, stressful thing happens to you, it's always bad and you're always dealing with adversity and negative consequences. And those events have some lingering damage. So this puts you at a greater risk of psychological and even physical health problems down the road," said Seery. "And it was just a very depressing picture."

But one day Seery came upon some research on a concept called "toughening." He explained, "It was this theoretical idea that being completely overwhelmed by negative, stressful things wasn't good. But it also theorized being totally sheltered shouldn't be optimal, either. There should be some amount of stress that gives you optimum psychological and physical well-being."

Seery found the toughening theory played out in animals. There was, for example, a study where scientists at Stanford stressed young squirrel monkeys. They removed them from their families once a week for ten weeks. When these monkeys grew up they were significantly more resilient and capable in the real world compared to their sheltered siblings. They were the leaders, the doers.

Seery wondered: Does the toughening phenomenon apply to humans?

Seery and his research team began a study. They asked people about the big stressors they'd faced in life. It was a perfectly ordinary group. There were 2,500 people who represented the broad spectrum of America. They were as young as 18 and as old as 101. They were half male and half female. They had the same racial makeup of the country. Some were rich while others were poor. This group was America.

The people regularly took online surveys in exchange for free Internet access. The surveys asked the people how many times they'd experienced stressors like a serious illness or financial difficulty, death of a loved one, violence, floods, earthquakes, and so on. It also asked them about their health and well-being. Are you depressed or anxious? Are you sick or in pain? How often do you have to go to the doctor, and how many prescription pills do you take? Are you happy?

What Seery found imploded the existing literature—and confirmed his notion.

Compared to the people who'd been sheltered their entire lives, "the people who'd faced some adversity reported better psychological well-being over the several years of the study," said Seery. "They had higher life satisfaction, and fewer psychological and physical symptoms. They were less likely to use prescription painkillers. They used healthcare services less. They were less likely to report their employment status as disabled." By facing some challenge but not an overwhelming amount, these people developed an internal capacity that left them more robust and resilient. They were better able to deal with new stresses they hadn't faced before, said Seery.

Seery knew he was onto something big. But he wondered whether he'd see similar results in a controlled environment. He brought a group of people into the lab and asked them how many trying events they'd had in their lives. He then had them stick their hand in a bucket of ice water and leave it there for as long as they could.

"The same relationship comes out," said Seery. "People report that the pain feels less intense if they have a history of some lifetime adversity. Not a high level, but, critically, not zero. Their mind is also less likely to go to a bad place during the experience. They also have fewer negative thoughts during and after the experience."

He's since done this with all kinds of stress-inducing tasks. He's put people through exams, had them give speeches in front of a big group, etc. His findings are consistent. "People who've gone through some adversity show a more positive response," he said. "They feel like the event is an exciting opportunity rather than a sense of overwhelming dread."

Based on findings like Seery's, there's a small but growing body of research that suggests people see the same effect by engineering big challenges. This new research looks at taking on epic outdoor tasks as a way to find the "physical, psychological, emotional, and spiritual" tools that Elliott wants to impart.

Take what teams of scientists based in New Zealand and the UK found. They combed through nearly 100 studies on the psychological impact of outdoor challenges. Their takeaway: Leaving the modern, sterile world and exposing ourselves to new stressors can help us develop the toughness that Seery is so passionate about. "Confronting risk, fear or danger produces optimal stress and discomfort, which in turn promotes outcomes such as improved self-esteem, character building, and psychological resilience," they wrote.

The desire in some of us to get out and test ourselves, one researcher believes, is "a sign of the times in which people are looking for a new way to . . . escape from an increasingly regulated and sanitized way of living." And something like a misogi might stoke something deep inside, because they incite stresses similar to the ones that men and women dealt with before all this comfort came at us, the researchers theorized.

This is why the scientists also believe that an outdoor test like a backcountry hunt or summiting a mountain can be better than more "contrived" challenges, like organized urban marathons or team sports.

I spoke about this with Douglas Fields, one of the country's leading neuroscientists. He's a senior investigator at the National Institutes of Health (NIH) who runs their department of neurocytology, which is the study of neurons.

He told me that when you undergo a new, stressful experience like misogi, you're transferring short-term memories into long-term memories—what just happened to you and what it led to, and what you should do next time you face a similar situation. "In general, this is because memory is about the future," said Fields. "We retain experiences that may be of survival value at another time."

I asked Seery specifically about misogi and mentioned the reports of Elliott, Parrish, and Korver. "That dovetails really nicely with how I think this stuff is working," said Seery. "There should be a common psychological process that leads to these benefits.

"If I develop fitness by swimming, I'm still going to be fit when I run," he continued. "I may not be a top-form runner, but the cardiovascular endurance will be there. Likewise with this toughening process. It should give me this internal capacity that leaves me better able to deal with many things."

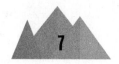

50. 70. OR 90.

ELLIOTT IS LIKE a misogi televangelist. He incited my interest in finding my own wild, terrifying, long-shot task. I wanted a misogi of my own. And so when Donnie called me with a proposition to do some serious edge surfing I was ready to jump.

"I'm going to Alaska for a month or so," he said. "It's going to be a massive, massive adventure. We'll go deep into the Arctic, hunting caribou. When we fly in there, you're going to think, 'This can't be real.' The land is wild and untouched for as far as you can see. The tundra is just so, so big. We'll time the trip to the great caribou migration. Thousands of caribou will be moving south, and it will be one of the most amazing things you'll ever see. There are grizzlies everywhere. Wolves, too. We'll climb ancient mountains and cross glacial rivers. We'll face violent storms. The Arctic is one of the most extreme places on earth. And we'll be utterly alone out there. If weather hits we could get stranded for days. . . ."

"Days?" I asked.

"Oh, yeah. Days . . ." He trailed off, then came back. "I want this to be a sincere, sincere adventure. We're going to see stuff every single day that will absolutely blow your mind. But we're going to have to be all in."

"OK," I told him. "I'm all in." We hung up and euphoria set in. For about two minutes.

I was then also blanketed with the realization that I was hazardously underprepared. Our Nevada trip was uncomfortable and while on it I longed deeply for the antiseptic comfort and safety of my modern life. But it was still well within the 50/50 range of me being able to complete it. This trip? Astoundingly more uncomfortable and risky.

I understood how Elliott must have felt standing atop the Grand Canyon's South Rim, looking over the 8,000-foot-deep gash in the ground separating him from the North Rim. Adventure and apprehension. Because another part of that same conversation with Donnie went like this:

"You realize this is going to be a lot more extreme and dangerous than the Nevada trip, right?" Donnie said.

"Yeah, I figured," I replied. "How much more extreme and dangerous?"

"Twenty times."

"Oh, I can handle that. I was afraid you were going to say fifty."

"Well, it might be fifty. Could be seventy . . . or ninety," said Donnie.

Ninety? Jesus. Sure, I'm an Eagle Scout. But the concepts of surviving killer weather, angry wildlife, and treacherous terrain; constructing emergency fires, lean-tos, and tourniquets; and tying the proper knot for every knot-tying scenario were deleted from my mind sometime in college after I discovered Evan Williams discount bourbon. Knots? I still tie my shoes bunny ears–style, the backup method for when your six-year-old isn't quite cognitively advanced enough for loop-swoop-and-pull.

"IN A PERFECTLY DESIGNED MISOGI, YOU GIVE IT EVERYTHING YOU HAVE AND YOU just finish it. Or maybe you just barely fail," Elliott told me. "To finish it with a lot left is not really doing it right. You want to explore what your potential is out on the edges."

And so it was that, six months before the bush plane was set to take off from that cold Kotzebue runway, I began an attempt to re-wild myself. With some preparation, I thought, I could take the odds that I make it through the entire trip from a long shot to a coin flip.

I recalled a conversation Donnie and I had in Nevada. "Let's say you wanted to start hunting tomorrow," he said as we were hiking to the peak of Cleve Creek Baldy, a roughly 11,000-foot vantage point where we planned to glass for elk. "It's all about preparing for a specific animal in a specific place at a specific time." Sure, he explained, you have to know how to draw a bow or fire a rifle. But you also need to learn the local hunting regulations, weather and land patterns, and everything about the animal's biology. How it leverages its strongest senses, travels across the land, and behaves under stress. Its sleep cycles, diet, and drives.

"You'll also have to build out the right gear system and calculate your food needs," said Donnie. The final step is the hunt, which won't be a walk in the woods. "Even seasoned hunters have about a twenty-five percent success rate," he tells me. "Think of how you'd move through the forest and behave if you knew a human was hunting you. That's how most big game have evolved to behave all day."

I needed to go from a desk-bound writer to a modern mountain man. And I had just a handful of months to cram for the exam.

I recalled the second rule of misogi and decided that a logical first principle should be to make it back alive. Which is how I found myself in the visitors' center of a nearby state park, sitting through an emergency wilderness medicine course. The two-day seminar promised to "teach me the wilderness medicine skills I'd need to recreate with confidence in the backcountry." It pitched itself as "ideal for individuals in remote locations." I'd learn how to deal with many of the horrors that could end up killing me. A broken spine or bashed-in skull (plane crash). Compound fractures and cavernous puncture wounds (cliff falls, gores). Hypothermia, lightning strikes, pulmonary edema (Alaskan weather and landscape). Et cetera.

The course was filled mostly with outdoor adventure guides, scoutmasters, camp counselors, and government wildlife biologists. For insurance purposes these people needed a stamped certificate confirming they'd taken the course. There were also a couple of retirees who arrived dressed as if the course were a stopover between a Hemingway safari and the summit of Mt. Everest. These gentlemen were wearing $1,300 worth of high-tech travel pants, shirts, and hats, oversize waterproof boots, and backpacks the size of a twelve-year-old that were fully loaded with Lord knows what. And I couldn't quite understand why these guys were taking the course. They made it clear that they knew everything about the wilderness and survival in it, a point they expressed by telling old-timey hearsay tales of outdoor horrors.

I suffered two days of the instructors and retirees preparing me for so many ways I could die or injure myself in the backcountry. But my biggest fear still hadn't been addressed. After the course, I approached one of the instructors, a minuscule, grinning, Minnesota-summer-camp-counselor-looking type. "What do we do in the event that a grizzly bear attacks?" I asked.

He gave me a disappointed-sounding response. "Yeah, we don't cover animal attacks in this course. There are just so many different animals that can attack you out there." Then he pepped up. "But you do now know how to dress gaping wounds! So if the bear were to attack, you could use what you learned here to stop the bleeding. . . ."

As he reviewed wound dressing, my mind drifted to a story my high school geometry teacher told me. The guy spent summers working on a fishing boat in Alaska, and he'd reward us with bear stories if we all turned in our homework. This particularly gruesome tale involved a young deckhand on a charter boat. The kid had spotted a massive blueberry bush on the shoreline and had gone to it to pick berries for guests. As the kid plucked, the boat's guests watched. Then they noticed activity on the bush's other side. A half-ton grizzly also thought blueberries from this particular bush seemed like a refreshing treat.

The two obliviously circled the bush. The tourists yelled at the kid. Their cries were swallowed by the wind and the river.

The bear and the kid picked on, obliviously converging. Until they met. The kid went saucer-eyed. The grizzly reared up on his hind legs, pulled back his massive paw—and slapped the kid's head clean off. Like a Little Leaguer hitting a baseball off a tee. Slapped off the kid's head. But, hey, I knew how to dress a puncture wound.

I got home and searched "what to do if a grizzly attacks," and landed on a page from the US National Park Service. Should a 1,000-pound grizzly decide to pick a fight with 170-pound me, the US government suggests I leave my pack on, fall facedown to the ground, play dead, and cover my neck with my hands. This technique, I assume, stalls the inevitable decapitation. And while I'm down there, I might want to spread my legs. This gives the bear a trickier time flipping me over so that he can then dig his four-inch claws directly into my soul.

Bears typically attack humans because we've inadvertently stumbled too close to their cubs, food, or territory. In which case, the bear usually stops short of killing and lets the person off with a mauling.

But all bets are off if the bear comes into my tent at night. That's the sign of a creature who craves human flesh. In that event, I'm to go full-on Sugar Ray Robinson, throwing haymakers, jabs, and uppercuts into the bear's face. This technique is useful, I was left to assume, because it injures your hands. The coroner then has enough evidence to confidently tell your family, "He went down with a fight." Assuming they recover the body.

But enough of the bear and what he's eating. I had to eat up there, too. Our crew wouldn't be surviving on hunted meat. "It could take weeks to find an animal, if we find one at all," Donnie explained. "We'll pack everything in."

Problem is, every ounce of food, clothing, and other gear in my pack would be more weight on my back. I didn't want to be walking out of the woods with leftovers, because they'd have weighed me down the entire trip. But I also had no intention of running out of food. This was a hunt and not a hunger strike.

Various calculators estimated I'd burn roughly 5,000 to 8,000 calories a day out there, which seemed like a lot of food to carry. Donnie explained that I'd be better off packing a livable amount of calories. Say, 1,800 to 2,500 a day. Extra energy could come from some of the excess weight on my body. "Oh, we'll be hungry," Donnie told me. "But we'll survive. I usually lose fifteen pounds every time I do a monthlong hunt."

For breakfast and lunch Donnie eats energy bars and calorie-dense items like nuts and dried fruit. No preparation needed. For dinner it's those freeze-dried backpacking meals that come in a pouch. Boiling water is poured directly into the pouch to "cook" the meal, sort of like instant ramen cups. These meals have a 30-year shelf life, weigh as much as a few Q-tips, and taste similar. I didn't love the food on the last trip with Donnie, but I understood the logic. So I'd also pack energy bars and freeze-dried backpacking meals. Maybe some trail mix, too. And, OK, a few candy bars. It was going to be a bland month, heavy on the preservatives and sugar.

Priority number two: Don't embarrass myself. I could surely apply the "Fake it till you make it" rule.

I didn't want to hold back the group or have them hear a single complaint from me. Unless my issue would somehow put us all in danger and break misogi rule number two. For example, "I'm cold." Nope. "I'm cold because I'm rather sure I have frostbite on my left foot and if the numbness spreads any higher up my leg you're probably going to have to carry me out of here." Reasonable. "I feel tired." No. "I feel tired and I think it's because I picked up hantavirus a few miles back. I'm afraid that just by looking at me you're going to catch this killer, too." Valid.

It was abundantly clear that I'd be cold, wet, and tired for most of the trip. Cold is a function of movement and layers. I'd be moving a lot, raising my temperature. And I'd happily carry extra layers to avoid frostbite and constant teeth chattering. But I couldn't pack just any clothes.

In fact, Donnie says an easy way to die in the wild is packing the wrong gear. First off, cotton will kill you. When wet, cotton becomes cold, and hypothermia sets in before you can say "I'm c-c-cold. . . . Do you think we're in t-t-trouble?"

"Wool and synthetics stay warm when wet, so you definitely want those for base layers," Donnie said. "Then you maybe want a wool sweater and socks. Definitely down pants and a down jacket with a hood. Also gloves and a hat. Then you want waterproof outer layers. We're going to wear the same shit every day. Bring an extra base layer and socks, in case those get wet. Otherwise, just one of everything."

For boots, Donnie put me in touch with a century-old German boot manufacturer called Hanwag. I checked the options on their website and found some designed for winter mountaineering excursions. One pair was rated warm down to -40 degrees Fahrenheit. The price was nearly $400. When I brought this up with my wife, she replied, "Well, how much would you pay to keep your toes?" More than $400. So the boots went into the cart.

I could and did buy my way into good gear and light food. But the one thing I couldn't sidestep with a credit card was being physically prepared. I would be repeatedly ascending and descending thousands of exposed vertical feet in search of an animal that I might have to eventually carry out in 100-pound sections. I had to rewild my workouts.

My typical workouts, like those of most modern people, are

basically to avoid drawing negative attention at the pool. Form over function.

But for this trip I'd require the skills humans had needed for millions of years in order to survive. The ability to climb steep mountain faces. Swiftly move in on an animal or escape a dangerous situation. Jump across a creek. Resist falls and rough ground. Persist while carrying heavy loads across long distances.

I emailed Dr. Doug Kechijian, an old friend who served in USAF Pararescue, in the Special Forces branch of the air force. When Navy SEALs or Army Rangers got injured in the field, Doug parachuted in to rescue them. He carried out missions in Iraq, Afghanistan, and the Horn of Africa, and one year was named an Outstanding Airman, which basically meant he was an MVP for the air force. When he was not saving lives in Fallujah, Doug was at Columbia University studying for a doctorate in physical therapy. Picture Captain America. Now add 40 IQ points.

Doug now helps US Special Forces soldiers and pros in every major sports league find the sweet spot where they can redline on a mission or in a game and avoid injury. He graciously agreed to lend his sporting wisdom to me, a gangly writer who considers his greatest athletic achievement to be holding the high score on various pop-a-shot arcade basketball games throughout the Las Vegas metro area.

"We need to turn you into a very physically versatile human being," he said. To do that, I'd do two weekly days of targeted strength training using kettlebells, barbells, and body weight. Think: movement patterns that the body was designed to do, like squatting, jumping, lunging, doing pull-ups, carrying, etc. Then I did a weekly day each of sprinting, walking uphill while wearing a 50-pound backpack, and hiking anywhere from 5 to 15 miles. I'd also start every workout with some drills to bulletproof the joints that are commonly injured out in the field. Ankles, knees, shoulders, etc. Roll an ankle out there, and it's a long hobble back to civilization. Unless the wolves find you early on.

This brought me closer to misogi rule number one—that 50/50 shot at making it to the other side.

Finding discomfort in Las Vegas was easy. All I had to do was walk into the desert. Hiking and running in the summer felt like exercising in a furnace. But these hikes and runs were also an oasis away from my daily life in the built environment. I'd toss on my gargantuan $400 boots (they needed breaking in, after all) and trudge through red rock canyons, black rock desert, Joshua tree forests, or piney highlands for a few hours each weekend. These natural environments acted like a pressure washer on my mind, clearing out the week's grime. Who needs to chat up a $100/hour therapist when there are long, quiet, empty trails waiting to be walked?

And my exercise in the heat delivered effects I couldn't get doing biceps curls and treadmill work as I watched *Dog the Bounty Hunter* down at some climate-controlled Mega Gym. According to scientists at the University of Oregon, people who exercised in a 100-degree room for ten days, for example, increased their fitness performance markers significantly more than a group who did the exact same workout in an air-conditioned room. The hot exercise caused "inexplicable changes to the heart's left ventricle." This can improve the heart's health and efficiency. Hot exercise also activates "heat shock proteins" and "BDNF." The former are inflammation fighters linked to living longer, while the latter is a chemical that promotes the survival and growth of neurons. BDNF might be protective against depression and Alzheimer's, according to the NIH.

I wasn't afraid to get a little creative. To get used to carrying heavy stuff all day, I'd throw on a 40- to 60-pound pack as I did chores around the house. Imagine: a grown man, vacuuming, folding laundry, and scrubbing toilets, all while loaded down like an infantry grunt. Or I'd toss on the pack and walk my dogs in my desert neighborhood while wearing my winter boots. I looked like a righteous asshole. Felt like one, too. But I'd rather look and feel like one in a

Las Vegas subdivision than perform like one once I got to the Arctic. Carrying weight over distance, I found, was a two-for-one that profoundly improved both my strength and endurance.

At night I read books and obscure old government reports about the environment where I was headed. Like Jack O'Connor's *The Big Game Animals of North America,* a book Donnie considers his bible. Or *A Sand County Almanac,* Aldo Leopold's opus on conservation science, policy, and ethics. Or scientific studies about the western Arctic caribou herd we'd be hunting. It was nice to experience the land and its challenges through the eyes of people who had gone and come back—many of them also writing nerds like me.

THE PREPARATION PROCESS QUICKLY REAFFIRMED MY NOTION THAT I SUCK AT NEW things. Wilderness savant I am not.

Trying to adopt survival skills, calculate calorie and gear requirements, move through all of the workouts, and understand complex ecological systems was a humbling and certainly bumbling experience.

There were workouts where I wanted to quit, frustrations as I tried to understand things I didn't, and serious dread that I was going to flub this whole thing and have the most miserable month of my life. If I even managed to make it that long.

Yet along the way I took comfort in the fact that I am not alone. We all suck at new things. But clumsily exiting our comfort zones offers way too many upsides to ignore.

Learning new skills—particularly the ones humans needed for millions of years that require us to use our mind and body—would stay with me beyond Alaska in a very Zen, the-path-is-the-goal type of way. There was all the new expertise I was picking up. But learning new skills is also one of the best ways to enhance awareness of the present moment, with no burning incense, Buddhist mantras, or meditation apps involved.

I needed only consider what I was doing before I started prepping for Alaska. I'd basically eaten the same meals, driven the same route to work, had the same conversations with coworkers, and come home to watch the same television for more than half a decade.

Scientists in the United Kingdom recently found that our brain has a trancelike "autopilot" or "sleepwalking" mode. Once we've done something over and over, our mind zones out of whatever old thing it's doing. Instead of being present and aware, we're far more likely to be lost somewhere inside our noggin. We're planning what we'll eat for dinner, wondering when the new season of that one show comes out, speculating about our office frenemy's salary. We live in a state of constant mental churn and meaningless chatter.

My months of preparation changed much of that. New situations kill the mental clutter. In newness we're forced into presence and focus. This is because we can't anticipate what to expect and how to respond, breaking the trance that leads to life in fast forward. Newness can even slow down our sense of time. This explains why time seemed slower when we were kids. Everything was new then and we were constantly learning.

Psychologist William James wrote about this in his 1890 work, *The Principles of Psychology:* "The same space of time seems shorter as we grow older. . . . In youth we may have an absolutely new experience, subjective or objective, every hour of the day. Apprehension is vivid, retentiveness strong, and our recollections of that time, like those of a time spent in rapid and interesting travel, are of something intricate, multitudinous, and long-drawn-out. But as each passing year converts some of this experience into automatic routine that we hardly note at all, the days and the weeks smooth themselves out in recollection to contentless units, and the years grow hollow and collapse."

A team of scientists in Israel confirmed James's notion in a series of six studies. They surveyed groups of people doing things that were either new or old to them. "In all studies," the scientists wrote, "we found that . . . people remember duration as being shorter on a routine activity than on a nonroutine activity."

This slowing down of time is something Parrish told me happens in misogi. "I become incredibly focused on the task at hand," he said. "When I look back on a misogi that was a few hours it will seem like days, because I remember every detail."

Additionally, stepping outside our comfort zone to learn useful skills that require both mind and body alters our brain's wiring on a deep level. This can increase our productivity and resilience against some diseases. Learning improves myelination, a process that essentially gives our nervous system a V-8 engine, creating stronger, more efficient nerve signals throughout our brain and body. Brains with more myelin are linked to improved performance across the board. Having too little of the stuff is connected to neurodegenerative diseases like Alzheimer's. Researchers at the University of Michigan, for example, found that dementia significantly dropped in people who dedicated more of their lives to learning. The fascinating part about that study was that dementia went down in the learners even though their rate of diabetes, a condition that increases the odds of developing dementia, went up. Which basically suggests that dedicating ourselves to learning new things could help offset some of our poor habits.

The day before I left, I was packing my refrigerator-size backpack. Wool layers, rain gear, boots, energy bars, freeze-dried meals, the works. I ran through a quick mental and physical checklist. I hadn't re-earned all my old Boy Scout badges, but I had pulled myself closer to the first and second rules of misogi.

I was leaner and stronger (ironically, the leaner part would actually hurt me once I began burning a massive amount of calories on the hunt). I could toss a 50-pound pack on my back and go pretty much until the authorities called me off. I'd also acquired a new library of natural knowledge, and found myself saying things to my wife like "Can you believe grizzly bears love moths? They'll eat forty thousand of them in a single day." Or "Did you know that if you nick an artery you can bleed out in just five minutes?"

I heaved the pack into the trunk of my wife's car. Then I headed to sleep in my warm, overstuffed bed for the very last time. She drove me to the airport early that morning, leaving me with a hug and a suggestion. "Don't get your head slapped off by a grizzly bear."

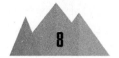

150 PEOPLE

"AS OUR AIRPLANES get smaller, our adventure gets bigger," Donnie told me as we planned for the trip. Escaping from an environment of comfort to one of discomfort is often a multistage process. This is because the average person is now vastly removed from the true wild. Getting to remote, unconnected, uncomfortable places like the Arctic requires traveling via a series of seemingly never-ending, successively smaller and more primitive modes of transportation. From jumbo jet to regional jet to bush plane or 4x4, and everything by boot thereafter.

I was anxious while walking through the Las Vegas airport. I couldn't figure out if my nerves were from all the impending flights or from committing to a 33-day trip off the grid with one pair of pants and two guys I only sort of knew. But it could also have been a symptom of the modern world I was leaving.

Satoshi Kanazawa, PhD, has spent much of his career considering what happens to humans in our overbuilt, overpopulated environments. He works at the London School of Economics as an evolutionary psychologist, which basically means he studies how our brains came to be and how our new world is changing them.

It's a topic worth understanding. And soon. We're increasingly jamming ourselves into cities. At the signing of the Declaration of

Independence only 5 percent of us were urbanites. By 1876, that number was still just 25 percent. But roughly 100 years ago we tipped to favor city living. Today, 84 percent of Americans live in cities and more are moving in. It's an odd trend.

According to a recent Gallup poll, only 12 percent of Americans actually *want* to live in a city (and that poll was taken before Covid-19). It seems many people may not have liked cities even when we started living in them, about 6,000 years ago. Before Christopher McCandless of *Into the Wild* fame headed into the Alaskan bush or Henry David Thoreau in 1845 trudged a half mile out into the woods and built a cabin at Walden Pond, there were scores of other men and women who exited civilization without fanfare and lived quietly, unseen and unheard. The world had the Desert Fathers and Mothers, monks who in the third century left civilization to live alone in the Egyptian desert. We had the Buddha, who around 540 BC bailed from the wealthy palace grounds to roam the open world as an ascetic. Even Jesus spent 40 days wandering the desert. He prayed and fasted, and resisted the temptations and promises of his modern world. This is why we give up beer and meat and we pray and fast during the 40 days of Lent.

A call to something untamed seems to exist deep inside humans. The same Gallup Poll found that most Americans today say they'd prefer to live out in the country or in a small country town. Which, considering our drive for survival, doesn't make a ton of logical sense, right? Darwin's theory of evolution rests on the idea that the traits that all species have are those that allow us to survive and procreate. Is living in the middle of nowhere really the best way to survive and spread DNA?

City living offers a far more comfortable and convenient life. Research shows that people who live in cities generally make more money (even after you adjust for the cost of living) and have more opportunities. They also have better access to sanitation services, healthcare, and nutritious food. And they can walk or take a quick cab ride to drugstores, supermarkets, emergency rooms, shrinks, restaurants, bars, concert venues, and museums. These are all places that provide survival benefits or help you find mates. Consider the collective thousands and thousands of bars, restaurants, drugstores, supermarkets, concert venues, museums, and doctors in Manhattan's 22 square miles.

Today it's possible to move into a big-city apartment and decide never to leave it. Literally never to walk back through the front door for years. It requires only a decent Internet connection to perform a job remotely, order food and groceries for delivery, and connect with telemedicine. This reality is already here. The Japanese government reports that there are half a million young Japanese who refuse to leave their bedrooms. They are called *hikikomori,* basically people who have sent themselves into an extended time-out. A third of them have spent more than seven years in self-isolation.

So why do we want to live in open spaces? What is it that, seemingly in competition with our drive to survive, cities are not giving us enough of? That's a question Kanazawa has spent years studying.

Some mental health researchers today call our concrete, sprawling environments "landscapes of despair." But the Industrial Revolution spurred a great migration into cities with the promise of secure jobs. We haven't turned back since. Yet, interestingly enough, money doesn't seem to overcome the rural/urban happiness gap. Studies show that even dirt-poor people who live in rural China report being happier than infinitely wealthier Chinese city-dwellers.

The notion that cities depress us is backed by numbers. People who live in cities are 21 percent more likely to suffer from anxiety and 39 percent more likely to suffer from depression than people who live in rural areas.

Two phenomena help explain this city/country happiness gap. The first is a rather curious number: 150. Consider the following set of figures:

148.4

150

150–200

125

Those numbers represent the population averages of hunter-gatherer tribes, Stone Age groups, villages in ancient Mesopotamia, and ancient Roman military legions.

A group of roughly 150 people or fewer seems to be an ideal community. It even has a name, Dunbar's number, after British anthropologist Robin Dunbar, who discovered it. As we evolved, groups of fewer than 150 people gave us enough resources to hunt, raise kids, share, and thrive.

When our groups exceed the limit, things tend to get weird. Managing more than 150 names and faces and all of the social narratives among them is a lot for our brains to process. Bigger societies are complicated and time-consuming (we have to develop government and laws), and that can burn us out.

This preference for a 150ish-person group size is likely wired into our brain from millions of years of evolution, and it still appears today. Now consider this series:

112.8

180

153.5

169

These numbers represent the average populations of today's Amish parishes in Pennsylvania, army companies in World War II, the personal network of the average American, and the number of real friends the average Facebook user reports having (despite a higher number of "Facebook Friends").

Dunbar explained it like this: "Human societies contained buried within them a natural grouping of around 150 people. . . . It's the number of people you would not feel embarrassed about joining uninvited for a drink if you happened to bump into them in a bar."

In his book *The Tipping Point,* author Malcolm Gladwell explained how this number impacts businesses. Take W.L. Gore & Associates, the company that makes the waterproof GORE-TEX fabric used in my boots, rain pants, and jacket. They discovered through trial and error that their office buildings with more than 150 employees had far more social problems. The solution? They built offices that hold no more than 150 people. The company credits this move to their success as a billion-dollar brand that is constantly named one of the nation's best companies to work for. It's interesting stuff. And making more money by hacking an office size is great and all. But Kanazawa is more interested in what Dunbar's number has to do with our desire to flee the city and live in the sticks.

He believes that we still prefer our original group sizes. Life in rural and small towns more closely mimics the environments we evolved in. The human population density of the world when we lived in hunter-gatherer communities was about 1 person for every 6 square miles. Compare that to Manhattan, which jams about 417,000 people into the same 6-square-mile space. Even midsize cities like Providence, Rhode Island, and Portland, Oregon, have 58,000 and 26,000 people per 6 square miles, respectively.

Therefore, "as population density becomes too high," Kanazawa wrote, "the human brain feels uneasy and uncomfortable, and such unease and discomfort may translate into reduced subjective well-being."

The discomfort cities provide can make it difficult for most of us to move our lives forward at a foundational level. Cities are fast-paced, overbuilt, overpopulated, overstimulating, no-effort environments— a dump truck's worth of psychic weight. Kanazawa calls his idea the Savanna Theory of Happiness, and the general rule of thumb is, the higher the population density wherever a person is, the less happy they'll likely be. Which may explain why a recent study by scientists at Harvard University found that New York City ended up dead last—318th of 318—in a ranking of the happiest American cities.

THE 108-PASSENGER JET TOOK ME TO SEATTLE, WHERE I MET UP WITH DONNIE AND William for the next flight to Anchorage. I found them sitting at the gate, looking like a grunge band that spends a lot of time in the woods and, apparently, hasn't been fed in a week. They both had long hair and beards and were dressed in flannel shirts and oversize Hanwag mountaineering boots. The two were scarfing Chex Mix and peanut butter M&Ms.

Both looked up at me with grins and started to chuckle. My own look was the result of what happens when a yuppie signs on for a stint in the woods. I had a couple days of stubble and was wearing outdoorsy yoga pants, a hoodie, and Crocs, which I planned to use as camp shoes. All of it was unworn until then.

"You ready?" asked Donnie. It was a fair question. "I guess we'll see," I replied. William offered up some M&Ms and I declined, because it was ten in the morning.

He eyed my bony frame. "Dude, you gotta eat," William said, rolling a half dozen more M&Ms into his mouth. "Yesterday I ate a Chipotle burrito and a Five Guys burger and fries. Doing my best to bulk up before the lean times, boys!" I was beginning to think that I should have packed on some extra pounds, so I grabbed a handful of Chex Mix.

Donnie leaned in to me. "We had to check fifteen bags," he said. That was packs, food, teepee, camera gear, gun, bow, and more. "So I made these fake media passes so we could get a media rate on our bags. It cost us three hundred dollars for all our stuff instead of fifteen hundred." He tossed me the media badge. "How does it look?"

It was the size of a credit card and hanging on a lanyard. It featured Donnie's mug and the logo of Sicmanta, his production company.

MEDIA was stamped across the top and there was a bar code at the bottom.

"What's the bar code?" I asked.

"Uhhh . . . we found it by searching 'bar code image' on the Internet," said Donnie.

Throughout my career I've had hundreds of media passes that have gotten me into locations with security as tight as that at the Pentagon. "Honestly, dude," I said. "This looks more legit than any media pass I've had." Soon we were called to board the four-hour flight to Anchorage.

Arriving at our ultimate destination, that northeastern dot on the map inside Ram Aviation, required two days of travel. So we spent a night in Anchorage. Our poor hotel shuttle driver looked at us like we just flipped off his grandmother when we told him that we had 16 heavy bags to load into his van.

We got a few hours' sleep and were back at Anchorage's Ted Stevens International Airport (does anyone else find it odd to name an airport after a senator who died in a plane crash?) before dawn for an Alaskan Airlines flight to Kotzebue.

The sun was rising from a gray blanket of clouds as the 124-passenger jet zoomed north. After an hour a neon-maroon band projected low across the horizon, which faded into a powder-blue sky. The only sign of land below was the thick white peak of Denali, the highest point in North America at 20,310 feet.

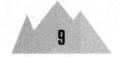

101 MILES

I SHOULD HAVE appreciated that flight into Kotzebue more than I did. I didn't think to savor the last bits of modern luxuries—multichannel TVs in the seatbacks, complimentary coffee, and, of course, running water and bathrooms. I'm thinking longingly of that cramped but comfortable seat as I'm thrust backward and Mike flies our Cessna off the ground and into the Arctic.

The Ram Aviation shack in Kotzebue shrinks as we climb to 359 feet in the air, then 678, then 993. We slowly gain elevation in sync with the mossy tundra as it ramps its way into the mountains. The rivers below, flanked by pipe-cleaner-shaped pines, are colored a milky emerald green. They bend and twist in a natural cursive across the taiga. The smell of the land rises to meet us. It's musk and earth, cold and clean.

William's forehead touches the glass as he sits in the plane's front passenger seat and stares down at the land like a bird of prey. He points out the grizzly, wolf, and caribou he's spotted below. The wind occasionally bounces us upward, drops us downward, or shoves us sideward. The engine powering the plane's single propeller is deafening.

I, meanwhile, am stuffed into the backseat and having something of an epiphany. My flight terror? Gone. This experience—the smell of the earth, the views, and the marvel that this freak little flying contraption is doing for us what used to take hunters a month on foot—is just too incredible. Fear is apparently a mindset often felt prior to experience.

I spend the flight in awe of the world below. In an hour Mike is cranking on levers and my ears are popping. The engine is whining hot and we're dropping elevation. And quickly. It's more a dive-bomb than a descent. We hit 1,900 feet. Then 1,700, then 1,600. The plane slams into a rocky but flat space of tundra.

The Cessna's tundra tires—bulbous, oversize low-pressure tires that absorb impact and allow for rough ground landings—ricochet us off the earth. We bounce, bounce, bounce to a stop. Then Mike is quickly tossing our gear out of the plane and mumbling that his plane is too big to land at our final destination. "Brian will be by sometime today to ferry you there," he says.

He takes off. William and I stand with our immense packs in the middle of this "runway," which is really just a flat, 100-yard stretch of cold, bumpy tundra.

From here the land dips and begins a long uphill trudge into mountains. It's a frost-covered gray-and-green world. The sky is washed in psychedelic smoky stratus and neon-white cumulus. The temperature has plummeted 20 degrees. It is 11:48 a.m. We are 101 miles from the nearest town.

Cell service disappeared about six inches out of Kotzebue and we've got nothing to do except wait for Brian. I'm at a loss for how to spend this unstimulated time, so I try asking William about his life in Maine. I quickly learn two things about him. The first: He's a man of few words—unless hunting is the topic of conversation. The second: He drops the F-bomb as often as most people say "the."

I learn that William's father, a 40-something Mainer, just yesterday arrowed "Bigfoot." Not the hairy folkloric ape creature who allegedly roams America's woodlands but a massive whitetail buck that William and his father first discovered six years ago. "There's this fuckin' island on the coast of Maine called Long Island. It's the largest island in the state without a full-time community on it," he says. William rowed out there one day and set up a trail camera. These cameras are triggered by motion and are often used by hunters and biologists. "We got some pictures of this big, big fuckin' buck," he says.

From there he and his dad spent thousands of hours on the island, learning about its landscape, restoring its habitat so deer could thrive, and scouting how this particular deer was living his life. "One day we came across this fuckin' gigantic footprint. So we named the deer Bigfoot." The deer will provide the family with clean meat for months.

William walks over to a grassy area to relieve himself on the frozen ground. I dive into my bag, looking to add another layer to the five I'm currently wearing. The Arctic cold is rapidly burrowing into my desert bones.

"Hey," William yells from the grass. "Look at this fuckin' thing." He's walking toward me, holding in his bare hand what appears to be a brown softball.

"Grizzly poop," he yells, bringing it to me. The turd is a voluminous wad flecked with fibers and seeds. "Fucker's been eating a lot of berries. Big poop means a big butthole means a big bear. The stuff's pretty dry, though," says William, crumbling the feces in his palm. "Hard to say when he was here." He drops the rest of the turd and it lands with a hollow thud. I note to avoid any future high-fives or handshakes.

After a few hours we hear a low whine. A white dot appears on the horizon. It's the plane Donnie left in. Brian is at its controls. He swoops, banks, and descends, hitting the earth to roll and stop within ten feet of us.

At six feet and 200-some-odd pounds, Brian in his plane looks like a dad who's wedged himself onto a kid's carnival ride. Piper Aviation from 1946 to 1948 built 3,760 of these PA-12s. Brian's is from the 1946 run. Roughly six years ago, some guy wrecked this particular PA-12. Brian bought the wreckage and rebuilt it to his exact specifications. He's upgraded the original 108-horsepower engine to one that'll produce 185 and added tundra tires instead of the also common floats or skis.

Most of these old PA-12s are still in operation. People up here often refer to them and other small Cub models as the taxicabs of the North. Their specialty is shuttling people and things into the wildest places where roads don't go. Few aircraft are as versatile and, generally, dependable. In 1947, for instance, two US Air Force officers, after a few rounds at the officers' club, bet they could fly two Super Cubs around the world. After four months and 22,500 miles of flying, they'd collected on that bet. The only mechanical issue they faced was a tailwheel damaged during a sketchy landing. Robust little aircraft, indeed. But, looking at Brian's plane, I find this claim impossible to believe.

If Mike's Cessna 180 is an empty can with wings, the PA-12—about as tall as me, 22 feet in length, with a 35-foot wingspan—is more like aviation's take on the fun-size candy bar. I approach it and notice tiny seams running up and down every couple inches of the craft. I touch a wing. The material covering it gives with my touch, flexing inward, like pressing on a taut piece of fabric.

I look at Brian with a "Did I break something?" look.

"The frame is wrapped in polyfiber, a plasticky fabric . . . basically duct tape," he says, and, seeing my look of alarm, continues. "But it's a special duct tape."

"Ohhh, OK, a *special* duct tape," I reply. "Ah, yes, that makes this vessel much more airworthy."

Brian chuckles and motions that we should get going. William grabs his pack, throws it into the back of the plane, and squeezes in. "I'll be back in a couple hours or so," Brian tells me. Three men and the gear would be too heavy for the 1,300-pound PA-12. It takes off, shuttling William to our final drop point and leaving me with myself and the big-butthole bear. No gun. No bow. The upside? If the bear attacks I won't have to worry about taking Mike's shitty plane home.

There is alone like "I need to be alone. I'm going to my room." And then there is the alone that I'm now experiencing, standing in the Arctic tundra with no human around me. I am surely the only person in this 6 square miles—or 12 or even 18. I've never experienced alone like this. I could scream and shout and hoot and holler and no one would hear. I could shoot up a flare or waft smoke signals into the great unknown and no one would see. I could get ass naked and do rain dances while singing Buck Owens at the top of my lungs and no one—not a one—would ever have a clue. This is the farthest away I've ever been from other people in my entire life.

It's an interesting paradox. Despite the fact that people today are rarely alone, we are increasingly lonely. The world is closing in on 8 billion people, a big bowl of human soup. People surround us at work, in the grocery store, during our commute, in our neighborhood. Even when we are by ourselves, we are often "with" the people who speak to us through our televisions, podcasts, or text messages. Yet nearly half of Americans say they're lonely, leading the US government to declare that we're facing a "loneliness epidemic."

The physical and mental health effects of this epidemic are substantial. Scientists at Brigham Young University found that it doesn't matter how old you are or how much money you have, being lonely increases your risk of dying in the next 7 years by 26 percent. Overall, it can shorten life by 15 years. That's equivalent to smoking half a pack of cigarettes a day. Good relationships are also, according to another study conducted over 80 years by researchers at Harvard, a key ingredient to happiness across your life span. Good relationships beat fortune and fame.

Which is why a growing wave of government reports and popular books, podcasts, and TED Talks are calling attention to the loneliness problem and giving advice on how to be less lonely. The messages are essentially "Get out there with a positive attitude, buddy! Do work at a coffee shop or library! Go to a party or concert! Join a softball team or running club! Talk to strangers!"

These methods are probably helpful and we should surely all work on building strong human bonds. But I'm also skeptical of the idea that, say, some Coors-swilling guy who plays shortstop for a softball team I signed up for could ever provide me with real emotional support or insight into myself.

I can't help but think that in today's increasingly hyperconnected and tribal society—where we define ourselves by the group or movement we belong to—it's not a bad idea to occasionally be alone. Removed from anyone. I'm talking about time with yourself, unidentified with anything. The Buddha, Lao-Tzu, Moses, Milton, Emerson, and many more have spoken highly of the benefits of solitude.

A growing field of scientists today think that these solitude-seekers were onto something. Building "the capacity to be alone" may be just as important for you as forging good relationships. "The capacity to be alone is essentially the ability to be alone with yourself and not feel uncomfortable or like you have to distract yourself," said Matthew Bowker, PhD, a professor of psychology at Medaille College.

The realization that I am in a state of supreme solitude is both unnerving and freeing. Unnerving because if the weather changes—and it does often and quickly out here—it could prevent Brian from landing the Super Cub and I'd be stranded for days. It's freeing because without anyone else around I'm completely unbeholden to any societal standards and there's no need to mold myself to the will of anyone else. I'm uncomfortable but untethered. The social narrative of how a man at 30-something should look, act, and carry himself just doesn't hold up when you remove society from the story.

Solitude is something people generally suck at. In a study conducted by scientists at the University of Virginia, a quarter of women and two-thirds of men chose to shock themselves rather than be alone with their thoughts. Imagine that. "You can either sit here without me in the room," said the researcher, "or I'll stand here with you, but you have to press this red button that sends high levels of electric voltage through your veins." And the participants responded with . . . "Hmmm, why don't you stay put and I'll just . . ." *Zap.*

Back on the tarmac in Kotzebue, Donnie told me about his first stint out of college working as a researcher for the Fish and Wildlife Service. They'd recruited a class of 24 college grads. Each had signed on to spend six months alone at a remote camp on the Yukon River delta collecting data.

"Nineteen from that group had dropped out and gone home in the first week," Donnie told me. "They'd get up there and just sort of freak out. You learn *a lot* about yourself over the six months that you're alone out there." Scientists at Miami University, Ohio, say that social media is making it even harder for people today to be alone. FOMO is spiking.

Our general discomfort with solitude may be due to how society frames it. Consider how we discipline children: time-out. Or how we punish prisoners: solitary confinement. This tradition, Bowker thinks, may have cued us to believe that normalcy is found through others and that solitude is punishment.

Covid-19 lockdowns were likely the first time that many people experienced extended alone time. Our unfamiliarity with being with ourselves is why University of Washington scientists predicted a loneliness-induced surge of clinical depression during the pandemic. This could explain why self-medication through eating, drinking, watching porn, and using drugs all spiked during quarantines, according to research.

I think about how I behave around others. I'm often wary of being unconnected for too long and my default behavior is to shape my personality to suit what other people will positively respond to. Sometimes it's like I live my life as a reaction to someone else.

"But there are a lot of great pleasures you can get out of the experience of being alone with yourself," said Bowker. In solitude you can find the unfiltered version of you. People often have break-throughs where they tap into how they truly feel about a topic and come to some new understanding about themselves, said Bowker. Then you can take your realizations out into the social world, he added: "Building the capacity to be alone probably makes your inter-actions with others richer. Because you're bringing to the relationship a person who's actually got stuff going on in the inside and isn't just a connector circuit that only thrives off of others."

Research backs solitude's healthy properties. It's been shown to im-prove productivity, creativity, empathy, and happiness, and decrease self-consciousness.

"Social connection is obviously critical," said Bowker. "But it can be dangerous if your social connections ever go away and you don't have yourself to fall back on. If you develop that capacity to be alone, then instead of feeling lonely, you could see solitude as an opportu-nity to have a meaningful and enjoyable time to get to know your-self a little better. To essentially build a relationship with yourself. I know this sounds cheesy, but it's critical. I think a goal we should all have is to try to transform feelings of loneliness into feelings of rich solitude."

As I stand in the quiet solitude, I go from feeling anxious to feel-ing unencumbered. Unaffected. It's a welcome change from all the humans and chaos of home. Occasional outdoor aloneness, the re-search of Kanazawa and others suggests, can be an antidote to the stress imposed by people-packed cities.

The silence is eventually interrupted by that low whine, and my solitude is severed. The Super Cub is nosediving into the tundra.

The plane bounces to a stop, and Brian hurriedly chucks my stuff into its hull. I jump in. The plane's frame is made of piping and the roof is clear Plexiglas. When Brian boards we're positioned like some lunatic Alaskan bobsled team. I'm sitting directly behind him with my knees up into his armpits. We launch into the air. The special duct tape trembles in the wind. Each gust has its way with the craft, pushing us up and down, side to side.

Brian points at the tundra. A herd of caribou is grazing a mossy slope. In 40 minutes I see two dots on a faraway mesa and we bank toward them. "This spot," Brian says, "is a bit of a tight landing. Hold on."

A wind gust pushes us backward as he banks. This whole scene feels comically deranged. That I'm traveling hundreds of feet above the ground at more than 100 miles an hour in a craft like this. That I'm about to be dumped in one of the most dangerous environments on earth. And that somehow, despite millions of years of human evolution telling me I should avoid risk, I'm enjoying the hell out of it. It's stress. But of a different type. A freeing stress.

‹70 MILES AN HOUR

THE WHEELS OF the Super Cub dribble onto a gravelly mesa half the size of a football field. The plane careens toward Donnie and William, who are waiting with tall backpacks and long grins. Once my gear is down, Brian is wheels up and back to Kotzebue. We have things to accomplish.

"The rules for surviving in the wild are shelter first, water second, food last," says Donnie. We have just one of the three. And it's the least important one at that. So we trek the rim of the bare mountain, looking for a decent place to pitch the teepee.

"Campsites are all about tradeoffs," Donnie says. "If we camp high on the mountain, we'll wake up in a spot where we can see caribou moving across the mountains and valleys and won't have to hike as far to a glassing knob each morning." We'll also be out of those valleys, which are where grizzly bears like to hunt. They hide in the alder thickets that flank the rivers and wait for some unsuspecting caribou or moose to wander down for a drink. Then they pounce and lay down a devastating attack.

"The downside of a higher campsite is that we'll be more exposed to the wind and a hike away from water and firewood," he says. And we'll also likely have to pitch the teepee on a slope, which means sleeping at awkward angles. Feet higher than head, left shoulder cantilevering off sleeping pad, and so forth.

We're in no rush to find a spot. Alaska law stipulates that you can't hunt on the same day you fly. It's a perfect piece of legislation designed to prevent hunters from searching for animals while buzzing above the land in a Super Cub plane. "That isn't hunting," Donnie says. "That's shopping." The law considers the act poaching. Particularly egregious poaching cases have been smacked with six-figure fines and a year in jail.

"Can you see them?" Donnie says, pointing to a northern hill. I squint and squint, scanning the mossy green hill. Nothing. "Look at the ridgeline," he says.

They appear. Twenty tiny white-and-brown dots on the light gray skyline. Caribou. "They can see us, too," says Donnie. "They've already seen us."

We pause and stare. Just below the ridge are 40 more dots. "How far is that hill?" I ask.

"Much farther than you think. This is a good sign, though. That's more than I've seen in entire trips up here."

As we walk, Donnie hears something and stops. "Water?" he says, listening. We look to the ground. It's covered in shale, moss, and big tufts of dry grass, called tundra tussocks.

There's a minuscule stream snaking between the tussocks. The flow is flanked by a fresh pile of caribou droppings and has caribou tracks running through it. William and Donnie both pick up a few caribou pellets, which are like oversize deer pellets. "This is fresh," says Donnie, pancaking the turd between his fingers. "They came through here recently for water." Then he bends down and fills his water bottle from the stream. He takes a long drink.

I, coming from a world where grocery stores offer 75 different varieties of bottled water, am wondering if this move is (a) wise or (b) a path into a gastric hellscape. "Is this water . . . ," I begin.

"Safe to drink? Oh, yeah," Donnie replies with the confidence of a man selling used cars. "I guess there's a small chance that you could get a parasite from it. So you get a little poopy pants for a day. Beats having to hike down to the river all the time."

I'm parched. So I fill my own bottle and take a drag. If one of us is going to catch a stomach bug, we all should. The water is cold and minerally and tastes like something you'd pay $5 for a liter of at Whole Foods. Then Donnie begins telling me that this pellet-flanked, hoofed-over water is likely cleaner than what comes out of the faucet at home. This tiny stream is one of the millions upon millions that boil up from the hillsides of the Arctic. The ground is in a constant state of thawing and freezing. This expands and contracts the land and forces water from it, filtering it. The Noatak River system, which we're smack in the middle of, is believed to be America's last remaining river system unaltered by humans.

We approach a semi-flat patch of grass on a ridge. "This place looks decent," says Donnie. "Here we'll be protected from the northeast winds for a few days. Then we'll move when they shift to southeast winds." We pitch the teepee, organize, and plan for tomorrow.

"We'll get up and have some coffee and breakfast. Then we'll move in toward that hill," says Donnie. Another benefit of higher camping spots: the view. The land unfurls forever and ever, revealing worn mountain after mountain in every direction.

We take to the teepee as the sun falls. "What do you want, boys?" Donnie says as he lights the backpacking stove and places a pot of water on it for boiling. He starts rummaging through our Mountain House dinner bags. "We've got sweet-and-sour pork. There's lasagna and spaghetti. We've got beef stew, chicken and dumplings. Beef stroganoff . . . oooh, William, you love beef stroganoff." He frisbees the bag at William.

We lie down to sleep before the sun disappears, around 9:30. The teepee's fabric walls begin to ripple slightly in the wind.

———

IT BEGINS AS A MUFFLED POP. MY EYES BURST OPEN FROM A DEEP SLEEP. *POP, POP, pop.* Like tiny firecrackers.

I pull my hand from the interior of my sleeping bag and bring it toward my face. The teepee is totally dark. My wristwatch's glowing hands tell me it's 2 a.m. I hear rustling. A light flicks on.

Donnie is sitting on the edge of his sleeping pad with his headlamp on. He looks at me, shining the light directly into my maladjusted eyes. I draw my hand over my face.

As my eyes adjust I can see the teepee fabric—waterproof ripstop—whipping abusively. The frost that's accumulated on it overnight is snowing onto everything. The entrance's metal zipper pull is like a sleigh bell, ringing as it dances back and forth. Donnie is saying something, but he's drowned out by the teepee's symphony.

I unzip my sleeping bag, then make a "one-second" hand gesture. I find my headlamp, sit, and lean toward Donnie.

"We're a sailboat right now," he yells. "The wind changed directions. We're completely exposed." Another light flicks on. William is up and sitting on the edge of his pad, too. "Fuck," he says.

"With the wind chill it's probably negative twenty out," yells Donnie.

The beauty of the teepee is that it has none of the annoyances of a tent. Ours has a max height of nearly 11 feet and leaves a 20- by 17-foot footprint. This means we can stand and move comfortably inside it. In low-roofed tents, anything and everything except sleep requires a person to contort him- or herself like a circus freak. The teepee also has no floor, which means we don't have to remove our boots each time we walk in and out or worry about dragging in wet gear. There is, indeed, a reason why many old cultures lived in teepees instead of tentlike structures.

There are also downsides. The teepee's height gives the wind more surface area to press against. If the structure goes airborne, it becomes a giant umbrella to be whisked somewhere into Russian airspace, leaving us and our gear exposed.

"Right now I'd guess the winds are about fifty miles an hour," says Donnie. "It should hold in this."

"Should," William says. "It's held in worse."

"Let's just try to go back to sleep," Donnie says. Which is like suggesting nap time during an air raid.

The frozen wind is infiltrating the teepee, swirling around and down my back. I burrow into my sleeping bag, don my beanie, and use my down vest like a scarf, leaving nothing exposed. The wind pushes into the side of the teepee, in turn pushing me with it. Like Mother Nature rocking me violently to sleep.

Fifteen minutes go by. Then 30. Then an hour. Then 90 minutes. The wind is constant. But by 5 a.m. the noise is picking up and the gusts are gaining speed. The inside of the teepee now sounds like a death-metal drum solo played inside a machine-gun range. I peer out of my bag. Donnie is up.

"These are hurricane-force winds now," he yells. "Gusts more than seventy miles an hour. We're asking too much of this thing." The southeast wall of the teepee is pushing into its aluminum main beam.

"Pack up and put on your down and rain gear," Donnie yells. If the teepee goes and our clothes, sleeping bags, and pads are exposed, they'll go sailing. An emergency takedown in the dark is too risky. So we sit and wait.

I'm feeling an all-encompassing body tightness as we sit around marinating in stress hormones and waiting for the weather to break our first rule of surviving the wild: having shelter. "I think this fuckin' main beam is going to snap," yells William.

In an hour, the sun begins to rise. "Let's try to break down," yells Donnie. I grab my pack and begin to unzip the entrance. The wind catches the door flap and rips it open. This tears up a stake and flings it 100 yards down the ridge.

We begin sprinting gear to the other side of the ridge. A protected, windless area is just 400 yards away, and so we do a few frantic hauls back and forth.

Then we all crowd around the pole inside the empty teepee. We'll have to lift it. But the wind is cranking into the fabric, driving the pole deep into the ground. Every hand wraps around the pole, and we all generate as much violent vertical force as we can. Nothing. Once more. Nothing.

"Fuck," says William.

"Move," says Donnie. He gets in close to the pole, feet flanking it. William and I surround him, grabbing free areas. Then Donnie is all back and legs. The beam rises an inch from the earth. I pull the pole's bottom and it falls horizontally, leaving us all draped in teepee fabric.

We move the shelter's remains to safety and William inspects the beam for damage. It's fine. But the wind drove the hollow beam into the ground with such force that it drilled through the rock on which it was placed. This created a perfectly round hockey puck of shale within.

Hours later we're sitting atop a faraway glassing knob, eyeing the hills for caribou. I think of the morning and how powerless we were in that weather. I can't help but chuckle. "What?" Donnie asks.

"This morning could have been pretty bad, huh?" I say.

He nods. "Brian told me about some hunters who were doing a five-day caribou hunt. For bear defense they brought rifles, .357 revolvers, shotguns, and an electric bear fence that attaches to a car battery," he says. "Everyone worries about bears. But weather is the shit that'll kill you."

And we've got 32 more days of it.

Then Donnie gets serious. "Yes, this morning could have been bad," he says. "But moments like that . . . you might find that they make everything else more colorful and more manageable."

PART TWO

Rediscover boredom. Ideally outside.

For minutes, hours, and days.

11 HOURS, 6 MINUTES

A CHOCOLATE CHIP Clif Bar has 250 calories. Its primary ingredient is "organic brown rice syrup," which I believe is a health-haloed euphemism for "sugar." The bar's creator, some guy named Gary, got the idea for it after a 175-mile bike ride and named the creation after his father, Clif. My Black Diamond down jacket "contains non-textile parts of animal origin." It must be machine-washed cold, gentle, without bleach, and tumbled dry on low heat. My backpack from Kifaru, a hunting gear company created in 1997 and based out of Colorado, was "sewn with pride in the USA by: HONG."

These are some of the things I learned while sitting on a hillside with nothing to do for 10 hours straight—no Internet, my only reading material the wrappers of energy bars and tags on outdoor gear.

Our days since the windy spectacle of day one have been routine. We wake, drink instant coffee, pack our stuff, and then hike to said hillside. Then we sit waiting for caribou herds to move into focus. Except the animals don't want to show. So we mostly just sit. Sometimes we talk. Sometimes we don't. This extended time in one spot, talking and not talking, staring at the same caribou-less landscape, has me wavering in and out of states of boredom I haven't experienced since, well, come to think of it, the last time I hunted with Donnie in Nevada.

To kill the time I've taken in the view. A lot. But my mind can only meditate on unchanged nature for so long. So I've also scrutinized the sales copy, nutritional profile, and ingredient list of every one of my energy bars. When that became dull I planned all my Christmas shopping. When that became dull I did more push-ups than I'd done during the entire prior year. When that became dull I came up with no fewer than 17 story ideas for some of the magazines I write for. Then I wrote some of this book in my little orange weatherproof notebook. Then I lay belly down and surveyed the ground. One square inch of Arctic earth contains microscopic spiders and weevils, long-dead Arctic poppy, white slivers of caribou moss, army-green moss, and neon lichen. These lichen, *Rhizocarpon geographicum,* can be roughly 8,600 years old, Donnie once read. That reminded me of a study in the journal *Global Change Biology,* which discovered that only 5 percent of all of the earth's land is unaltered by humans. The untouched places exist in the boreal forests, taigas, and tundras of the northernmost latitudes. These very patches of northern ground where we've been sitting, walking, and sleeping have likely never been sat, walked, or slept on by humans. (That thought killed a good ten minutes.)

This morning we're slowly shuffling around camp and stuffing gear and food into our bags as we discuss which hills to sit atop and what to do about these elusive caribou. Each fall the 250,000-strong Western Arctic caribou herd hoofs its way south from their summer calving grounds far north on the Beaufort Sea to their wintering grounds on the Seward Peninsula. It's a roughly 400-mile journey down an eons-old natural highway. We're at a location about 150 miles along this great migration route, and the caribou should be coming through like L.A. traffic.

"We see hundreds on the day we land and can't hunt, and none the past few days," says William. "Of course it works out like that."

"This game is never easy," says Donnie. "We just have to be patient and positive." And really good at dealing with boredom, apparently. I'm thinking about what I can do to manage today's forthcoming mental malaise when Donnie's eyes leave William and me. He squints at a hill beyond us. "Wait," he says, "Wait . . . Holy shit."

William and I spin around. We didn't have to be patient for long. About 30 caribou have emerged on a hillside about half a mile from camp. They're all leading uphill with their antlers as they chomp down tundra moss. Among them is a bull the size of a 1960s Buick.

Donnie brings the binoculars to his eyes. "Boys, that one in the back of the herd is definitely a shooter," he says. "Shooter" is the term he and William use for any caribou that they'd be willing to . . . shoot. Alaskan law states that we can only hunt antlered males. Maintaining about 40 males for every 100 females is ideal for the health of the ecosystem. The law does not, however, say anything about how old that antlered male must be. We'll only harvest caribou that are on the last of their 8 to 12 years of life.

"Oh, man," Donnie says, pulling the binoculars from his face and tossing them to William. "He's a handsome, handsome old boy."

William looks toward the herd. "Oh yeah . . . oh yeah. He's fuckin' ancient," he says, and hands me the binoculars. The animal is thick like a pig, with long thin legs. His coarse hair begins brown on his face, transitions to white at his neck, and then darkens back into auburn across his body. Antlers on an old animal like him are something to behold. His are massive question marks reaching high into the fog. They have long, flame-shaped fingers expanding everywhichway off the tops. Bisecting his face is an antler the shape of a flattened baseball mitt, called a "shovel."

Of all the animals in the North American Cervidae family, caribou have the largest antlers in relation to their body size—bigger than moose, deer, or elk. They generally form a big open C-shape, with elongated, conical points coming off the tops and bottoms. And they also have a distinct shovel-shaped piece that grows off the front of either their left or right antler and shoots out over their face. Caribou use it in winter to dig through snow so they can eat the frozen plants hibernating below.

Caribou antlers can grow longer than four feet. This is amazing in itself. But it's even more incredible when you consider that caribou, like all Cervidae, shed their antlers each year and regrow them in a few months. Antler is, in fact, one of the fastest-growing tissues on earth. It forms in rigid, staggered fibers that are able to slide past one another on impact. This makes it one of the lightest, strongest substances on earth. Antlers are such a feat of engineering that scientists today are researching how they can mimic antler construction to create stronger, lighter products.

"OK," I say, after taking a moment to marvel at the animal. "What's our play here?"

"We're going to sweep around that hill the herd is working their way up," says Donnie as he uses his finger to draw a map on his open palm. "Then we'll post up on the hill across from it and hopefully catch them as they eat their way northward."

Then we're like soldiers at the sound of a mortar, all sprinting into the teepee to hurriedly shove the rest of our gear into our packs. I lash the rifle onto my bag as Donnie grabs a handful of rounds. I've been carrying the long, cold weapon this whole excursion. Until now it's felt like something of a prop. A slight tension sets into my chest as I realize that I might have to actually . . . use it.

We begin fast-walking away from the herd and cut downhill to where the caribou can't see us. From here we can see our destination: a hillside about three miles away. We start hiking as the frozen wind thrusts itself into our faces.

Finally, I think. *Action! Movement! No more boredom!*

THANKS TO TECHNOLOGY, I RARELY LET MY MIND WANDER. I ALWAYS HAVE A PHONE, TV, computer, or other digital device to attend to. The average

American each day touches his phone 2,617 times and spends 2 hours and 30 minutes staring at the small screen. If that seems gross, the study also identified a large group of "heavy users" who spent more than 4 hours a day on their phones. In a course I teach as a professor at the University of Nevada Las Vegas (UNLV), I have students check their phone's screen-time data. One student averaged 7 hours and 44 minutes a day. Another racked up 8 hours and 32 minutes daily. "Why?" I asked.

"'Cuz YouTube," the student replied.

My own habits? I typically average three daily hours. Gross.

Let's say I live 60 more years and keep up that pace. I'll have spent seven and a half years of the rest of my life looking at my phone. And let's face it: I'm not using the device to read literary classics, learn a new language, or wire money to widows and orphans. I'm using my phone to google the answer to any half-baked question that leaks out of my gray matter or watch the social media mobs decry whatever they've deemed the "microaggression" of the day. Or, you know, "'Cuz YouTube."*

Smartphones are not only stealing our boredom, they are also shoving society dangerously close to, as screenwriter and satirist Mike Judge calls it, "idiocracy" status.

For 2.5 million years, or about 100,000 generations, we had nothing digital in our lives. Now the average person spends 11 hours and 6 minutes a day using digital media. That's from cellphones, TV, audio, and computers. Smartphones only stand out because they're newer, actively steal our attention with notifications, and are accessible at anytime. But the average person still spends double the time watching TV than they do on their smartphone.

So all these measures that help us "break up with our phone" are great. Unless we swap our phone time to binge-watch some Netflix

---

* One video on YouTube worth watching and rewatching is *Who We Are*, Donnie's seven-minute masterpiece on his hunting ethic.

series or surf the Internet on our laptop. That's like quitting smoking Marlboro Reds to pick up chewing Red Man.

Boredom is indeed dead. And one scientist way up north in Ontario, Canada, is discovering that this is bad. A type of bad that's infected us all. He believes that our collective lack of boredom is not only burning us out and leading to some ill mental health effects, but also muting what boredom is trying to tell us about our mind, emotions, ideas, wants, and needs.

PICTURE A ROADIE FOR AC/DC. NOW PUT HIM IN A CANADIAN NEUROSCIENCE LAB.

Congrats, you have James Danckert, a long-haired Aussie who's been studying the human brain on boredom at the University of Waterloo for nearly two decades. His path into the topic was guided by broken glass and bent steel.

Danckert was 19 when his older brother suffered a serious brain injury in a car accident. "During my brother's recovery and the years that followed, it was evident that he had changed," said Danckert. "He would tell me that he got bored a lot, and he was getting bored doing things that he used to really enjoy prior to his car accident."

So Danckert, then a university student, became obsessed with the brain and the state of boredom. "I didn't have any notions of fixing my brother. But I became fascinated by the notion that boredom is not a social or cultural thing. It's something within the brain that processes pleasure, reward, engagement, whatever you want to call it."

And he had the realization that boredom can be pretty damn uncomfortable no matter how healthy you are. "I hated being bored," he said. "I never liked the feeling of experiencing it."

Danckert isn't the only one to feel both fascination and loathing for the state of boredom. Philosopher Martin Heidegger accused boredom of being "an insidious creature." Søren Kierkegaard called boredom "the root of all evil." Psychologist Erich Fromm considered it "one of life's great tortures, a hallmark of Hell." Attitudes don't seem to be getting any better in today's world. So many podcasts feature some "top performer" or "life-hacker" guest. They tell us doing nothing is akin to dying and that we must therefore perform all of their complicated rituals to achieve optimum focus and machine-like productivity.

But new science is revealing that those otherwise brilliant philosophers and today's productivity gurus are clueless about boredom's potential, said Danckert. Sure, it doesn't feel great. "But boredom is neither good nor bad," he said. "How you respond to it is what can make it good or bad." The man knows this because he's been inside the human mind, searching for what areas of the brain are at work when a person is feeling the discomfort of boredom.

He recruited some volunteers and put them into a neuroimaging scanner. "Then we induced those people into a mood of being bored," he said. "We had them watch two guys hanging laundry for eight minutes. And . . . yeah, it succeeds in making people bored shitless."

When Danckert looked at the neuroimages of the bored people, he found that their insular cortex had deactivated. "That part of the brain is important for processing information that you think is relevant for your goals right now," said Danckert. "So it's down-regulated because there is nothing in that video that is important to your goals."

People are then spurred to do something about their boredom. "Tolstoy had this great quote in *Anna Karenina* that says boredom is a 'desire for desires,'" said Danckert. "So boredom is a motivational state."

In the study, Danckert also showed in what direction the brain goes when you're doing a whole lot of nothing. When the participants were bored, a part of their brains called the "default mode network" fired on. It's a network of brain regions that activates when we're unfocused, when our mind is off and wandering. "Default mode network" is an annoyingly dense term. For simplicity's sake I'll call it "unfocused mode."

Our brains essentially have two modes, focused and unfocused.

Focused mode is a mind at attention. It's on when we're processing outside information, completing a task, checking our cellphone, watching TV, listening to a podcast, having a conversation, or anything else that requires us to attend to the outside world.

Unfocused mode occurs when we're not paying attention. It's inward mind-wandering, a rest state that restores and rebuilds the resources needed to work better and more efficiently in the focused state. Time in unfocused mode is critical to get shit done, tap into creativity, process complicated information, and more.

The 11 hours and 6 minutes of attention we're handing over to digital media isn't free. It's all spent in focused mode. Think of this focused state like lifting a weight, and the unfocused state like resting. When we kill boredom by burying our minds in a phone, TV, or computer, our brain is putting forth a shocking amount of effort. Like trying to do rep after rep after rep of an exercise, our attention eventually tires when we overwork it. Modern life overworks the hell out of our brains.

Our collective lack of boredom may be causing us to reach near-crisis levels of mental fatigue. Research shows that the onslaught of screen-based media has created Americans who are "increasingly picky, impatient, distracted, and demanding," as one media analyst put it. These terms fall under the umbrella of "insufferable." And overworked, undermaintained minds are linked to depression, life dissatisfaction, the perception that life goes by quicker, and increasingly missing the beauty of life that only presents itself when we allow our mind to wander and be aware of something other than a screen.

Danckert explained that to understand why humans developed the capacity for boredom, we need to picture two cavemen. Each is picking berries from a separate bush three hours before sundown. In the scenario the first caveman is able to get bored. The second caveman is not.

The first caveman starts picking berries from his bush. But as he picks more and more berries, it takes more effort to find and reach the remaining berries. They're in hard-to-see-and-reach areas of the bush. Because he's receiving fewer berries for his time, the uncomfortable sensation of boredom kicks in. It compels him to find another bush and pick its most convenient berries. He repeats the process, picking the quickest-to-pick berries from a handful of different bushes. In an hour, he has two pounds of berries. And, with two hours of light left, he manages to spear a small kudu.

The second caveman quickly picks his bush's easiest-to-pick berries. But he doesn't have the cue of boredom. So he keeps picking from the same bush. This means he has to begin looking and reaching deep into the bush to find more berries. The amount of berries he's getting is tanking. But, hey, this is thrilling work when he doesn't have boredom telling him it's actually an incredibly inefficient use of his time. By sundown he's picked the entire bush and has his two pounds of berries.

At the end of the day, caveman one's family is eating kudu for dinner and berries for dessert. Caveman two's family is rationing out berries, trying to ignore how hungry they are. Before bed, caveman one will again experience the magic of boredom. His mind begins to wander. It rests and resets, planning how to hunt the next day, how to improve his family's life, or how to help his neighbor more efficiently pick berries.

The way we dealt with boredom before we began surrounding ourselves in constant comfort delivered benefits that are essential for our brain health, productivity, personal sanity, and sense of meaning. But there's been a cosmic shift in boredom. The way we now deal with it is "like junk food for your mind," said Danckert.

Sitting on that hill over the past days, I found my mind swinging between focused and unfocused mode. I'd notice something about the landscape, like a bevy of ptarmigan or the nuances of the Arctic light. Then the entertainment of the natural world would wear off and my mind would go searching for something more satisfying.

I'd go inward, thinking of, say, ways I could be a better husband. When the ideas stopped flowing, when the return on my time had worn thin, my mind would go somewhere else. Thinking of friends I needed to call, and on and on, to new places far more interesting or productive than anything I've found inside an app.

And so it was that on this march for that big bull, I actually found myself missing boredom. The opportunity to mind-wander. To be unfocused. Because in this moment the Arctic was, in fact, putting me in a dangerous position that forced me to focus entirely outward. Exceedingly outward. Down at the ground, scrutinizing every step. If my mind were to trail off, things weren't going to end well.

KNOWING WHERE TO GO ON THE TUNDRA IS ONE THING. BUT ACTUALLY GETTING there is quite another. The ground is like some mad landscape out of a Dr. Seuss children's book. Picture a massive, undulating, dull green mattress covered in partially inflated, weed-covered basketballs. The mattress is composed of dirt that exists in an ice-cream-like state, spongy layers of dense moss, mucky swamp, and partially frozen moving water. These soft layers sap energy from each of your footsteps.

There are also the aforementioned basketballs, known as tundra tussocks. They are spheres of densely wound cotton grass that sit like infinite warts atop the ground. They're spaced around 12 to 18 inches apart from each other in all directions and can live for more than 100 years.

So I've got a choice. I can step from tussock to tussock. But, given their bulbous shape and pliability, one awkward step can send my weight careening over my feet. This may snap an ankle or knee joint and leave me a crippled klutz who is miles from anywhere a rescue plane could ever land. Or I can walk on the mattress between them. Do that and each step takes more effort. The ground is cushiony, and I'll have to high-step around all the tussocks and be more likely to soak or muck out my boots. But at least my steps are less likely to result in grave disability. Either way, I'm spending the entirety of the hike face to the ground, heart rate cranked, focused on my foot placement like it's a bet on my ability to walk.

Occasionally we'll find an animal trail to follow. Those can be flat and firm one moment and the next have us scrambling across the side of one of the mountains as tile-like pieces of shale skim us downhill. There I slip about every 100th step.

After two hours of head-down hiking, we believe the caribou are on the other side of a knob we've reached. We all kneel down and plan, trying to anticipate what this herd has done and will do. "We need to get eyes on them," says Donnie. "Stay here." He belly-crawls to the top of the knob and lifts the binoculars to his face.

Then he's quickly turning and shimmying across the tussocks right back at us. "They're down there. We should hurry and swing around to that cliff area," he says, all stirred up and pointing to a craggy hilltop about a mile away. "The wind is at our backs now, which is bad. But if they keep eating up the hill and we can get there, we'll be blocked from the wind and in a perfect position."

We crouch and move quickly as the wind hits 15 to 25 miles an hour and streams through our jackets and dries our faces. In Patagonia they call this La Escoba de Dios, the Broom of God, a wind that constantly sweeps the landscape clean.

Wind is either a hunter's asset or liability. For any success, we must be downwind of the animal, its scent being pushed to us and not the other way around. Caribou can not only sniff out predators from hundreds and hundreds of feet away but also use scent as a warning. Their ankles have scent glands. When one senses danger, he'll rear up on his hind legs and pepper-spray the herd with a special smell that sends a DEFCON warning. The alert will send them all sprinting for higher ground.

I haven't showered or changed clothes in days. I can only hope that this wind isn't picking up whatever noxious pheromones are wafting off me and streaming them into the noses of the caribou.

THE EFFECTS OF OUR OVERSTIMULATED, STRESS-AVERSE SOCIETY ARE MOUNTING.
More than half of adults said they were under "high stress" in 2017.
Anxiety grew by 39 percent in a recent one-year period. Attention
spans fell by 33 percent from 2000 to 2015. Depression diagnoses are
up 33 percent since 2013.

Dr. Judson Brewer, a professor of psychiatry at Brown University Medical School, studies addiction, deals with many addicts, and
develops methods to get them better. He's particularly interested in
the tie between screen time and our growing mental health issues. "I
wouldn't pin this on mobile technology one hundred percent," said
Brewer. "But I'd say it's ninety percent due to it."

So it's no wonder Steve Jobs famously wouldn't let his children
use the iPad. He's not the only tech guru who questioned what he
was pushing. A massive swell of Silicon Valley workers who develop
mobile tech and apps don't allow themselves or their kids to use the
Valley's products. One former Facebook exec told the *New York Times*
that she is "convinced the devil lives in our phones." Another said that
Silicon Valley tools are "ripping apart the social fabric of society."

Picture yourself at a Target, Costco, or really any retail store. You
take a product to the checkout counter and hand it to the clerk. She
rings you up. And then she points to your purchase, locks eyes with
you, and whispers gravely, "I am convinced the devil lives in this."
Would you (a) assume this was the beginning of a real-life horror
film in which you are the main character or (b) buy the product and
use it hours each day? Apparently we all go with (b).

For one, these tools can be leveraged for evil—hi, Russia—and
for another . . . these tools can be leveraged for evil. Apps are engineered around Fogg's Behavior Model. If that sounds like something
menacing that was cooked up in a mind-control lab, that's because
it . . . kind of was? "Three elements must converge at the same moment for a behavior to occur: Motivation, Ability, and a Prompt,"

wrote Stanford psychologist B. J. Fogg. It's a formula leveraged by smartphone apps to make them behave like crack cocaine for our attention, and was created by scientists at Stanford's euphemistically named Behavior Design Lab.

Fogg originally designed the behavior model for good. Say, using phones to get people to quit a bad behavior, like smoking. But upon the advent of the iPhone, he had students begin applying the model to mobile tech.

One of his 2007 classes, now known as the Facebook Class, built apps that integrated with Facebook. Over one semester they grabbed 16 million users and a million dollars in ad revenue. Those students went on to work at companies like Facebook, Uber, Twitter, and more—and they took Fogg's Behavior Model with them.

Take, for example, someone posting a selfie to Instagram. The person is clearly *motivated* to want to know how her followers will react to her photo. Then Instagram *triggers* her with a notification that someone has commented on her photo. Did they like it, or is it a snarky comment? She then has the *ability* to check the comment immediately. She can't not open her phone.

And then, of course, she ends up checking her likes and comments all day, each time falling into an Instagram blackout where she scrolls her feed to find perfectly edited photos from a frenemy or conspiratorial posts from some glue sniffer she knew back in high school. All the while she's also seeing a ton of advertising, which is why Mark Zuckerberg is worth about $100 billion. A rule: If you're not paying for a digital service, YOU are what the company sells. The corporation games the system to take as much of your attention as it can in order to sell it to the highest advertorial bidder.

Still today, the latest round of whiz kids sit around the Behavior Design Lab figuring out how to compel us to engage with apps so that we'll see more ads. And these kids are damn good at what they do. Take, for example, the fact that notifications in Twitter and likes on Instagram take a few seconds to show up when you open the app.

That's no accident. That brief moment is like waiting for the wheels on a slot machine to line up. It leverages the same biological mechanisms to keep us coming back. These Silicon Valley savants have big data telling them exactly what tricks will grab us, and morons like me don't stand a chance.

Some researchers say "addictive" is too strong a term for cellphones. Because the drive to constantly check email and notifications is experienced differently than, say, the drive to drink or take drugs. But, as a person who knows addiction, I can tell you that the obsessive pull of my pinging phone sometimes feels just like the allure of a neon-signed honky-tonk. There's this famous line in recovery: "Try to drink and stop abruptly. Try it more than once." OK, try to ignore the beeping cellphone. Try it more than once.

"I like the simple definition of addiction being 'continued use despite adverse consequences,'" said Brewer. One good sign that I had a drinking problem was that most of my problems were caused by my drinking. And yet I found myself powerless to the pull of barrooms. For Brewer, it's no shock that many people are addicted to "the slot machines in our pockets," as he called them. Evolution says we should be.

"There's this evolutionary survival process we developed to help us remember where food is, so we wouldn't starve," Brewer told me. We'd see food, eat it, and then our stomach would signal to our brain to release a shot of dopamine, a feel-good brain chemical, he said. It's the same chemical that spurts out when people do drugs like cocaine or ecstasy, eat a gluttonous meal, have sex, gamble, or do anything else pleasurable. It's also a three-stepper.

"There's a trigger, a behavior, and a reward," said Brewer. "But this brain process can get hijacked in the modern day. The trigger instead of food is boredom. And the behavior is going on YouTube or checking our news feed or Instagram. And that distracts us from the boredom. We become excited and get a hit of dopamine, which is a reward.

"The paradox is that these mechanisms that helped keep us alive are now hurting our health," he explained. "We have less tolerance for distress. If we feel something unpleasant, like boredom, typically we would have to just be with that unpleasantness, and then we'd find a productive outlet. But we don't have to do that anymore. We can use our phone to distract ourselves." Or, as Danckert put it, we simply consume more "junk food for the mind."

Each time we reflexively take out our phone or turn on a computer or TV to kill boredom, it attaches another tiny anchor to our stress tolerance, dragging it lower. Scientists at Oregon State University found that daily stressors like lines and waits can improve our resistance to some brain diseases if we simply suffer through them and shrug them off. More of these everyday stressors are actually better for our brain.

THERE'S ANOTHER MASSIVE BENEFIT TO BOREDOM BEYOND MAKING US MORE PSY-chologically robust and resilient. Finding a different outlet for boredom also lets us tap into creativity.

In an interview with Bill Simmons, the acclaimed and prolific screenwriter Aaron Sorkin summed up this phenomenon when he talked about the first time he ever wrote for fun: "It was one of those nights in New York where it feels like everyone has been invited to a party you weren't invited to. I didn't have three dollars in my pocket. In [my] apartment was a semiautomatic typewriter. Electric keys and a manual return. The TV was broken, the stereo was broken. The only thing to do was to put a piece of paper in that typewriter and to start typing. Pure boredom. It was the first time I wrote for fun . . . and I loved it. I stayed up all night writing and I feel like that night has never ended."

Sorkin's takeaway is that we should learn to deal with boredom, and then discover ways to overcome it that are more productive and creative than watching a YouTube video or scrolling through Instagram.

Research from the 1950s backs up Sorkin's connection between boredom and creativity. One team of UK researchers had people do something astoundingly boring: read a phone book for 15 minutes.

The bored people then took a standardized creativity test, like coming up with odd uses for a Styrofoam cup, and the Remote Associates Test (RAT), where three words are thrown out and we have to figure out their common denominator (e.g., call + pay + line = phone; motion + poke + down = slow). Compared to a nonbored group, the bored people gave significantly more answers on both tests, and the answers were also considerably more creative. Other studies have found the same phenomenon. (Except in those studies the researchers bored people by having them watch a screensaver or separate a pile of beans by color.)

"But now people want to say that boredom *makes* you more creative," said Danckert. "I call bullshit on that. Boredom doesn't make you more creative. It just tells you 'do something!'" And when that "something" is letting our mind revive unfocused mode—or sitting down to write a screenplay—rather than blanketing it with the exact same media that everyone else is consuming, we begin to think, quite literally, on a different wavelength. That's what creativity requires.

Ellis Paul Torrance was an American psychologist. In the 1950s he noticed something off-target about American classrooms. Teachers tended to prefer the subdued, book-smart kids. They didn't much care for the kids who had tons of energy and big ideas; kids who'd think up odd interpretations of readings, invent excuses for why they didn't do their homework, and morph into mad scientists every lab day. The system deemed these kids "bad." But Torrance felt they were misunderstood. Because if a problem comes up in the real world, all the book-smart kids look for an answer in . . . a book. But what if the answer isn't in a book? Then a person needs to get creative.

So he devoted his life to studying creativity and what it's good for. In 1958 he developed the Torrance Test of Creative Thinking, and it's since become the gold standard for gauging creativity. Torrance had a large group of children in the Minnesota public school system take the exam. It includes exercises like showing a kid a toy and asking her, "How would you improve this toy to make it more fun?"

Torrance analyzed all the kids' scores. He then tracked every accomplishment the kids earned across their lives, until he died in 2003, when his colleagues took on the job. If one of the kids wrote a book, he'd mark it. Kid founded a business? Mark it. Kid submitted a patent? Mark it. Every achievement was logged. What he found raises big questions about how we judge intelligence.

The kids who came up with more, better ideas in the initial test were the ones who became the most accomplished adults. They were successful inventors and architects, CEOs and college presidents, authors and diplomats, and so on. Torrance testing, in fact, smokes IQ testing. A recent study of the kids in Torrance's study found that creativity was a threefold better predictor of much of the students' accomplishments compared to their IQ scores.

And now we've killed off one of the main drivers of creativity: mind-wandering. The result? A researcher at the University of William and Mary analyzed 300,000 Torrance Test scores since the 1950s. She found that the creativity scores began to nosedive in 1990, leading her to conclude that we're now facing a "creativity crisis."

The scientist blames our hurried, overscheduled lives and "ever increasing amounts of [time] interacting with electronic entertainment devices." And that's bad news. Particularly when we consider that creativity is a critical skill in today's economy, where most of us work with our brains rather than our brawn.

And so, despite what productivity gurus will have us believe, the key to improving productivity and performance might be to occasionally do nothing at all. Or, at least, not dive into a screen. It prompts us to think distinctly, in a way that delivers more original ideas. Even the god of Silicon Valley bought in. Steve Jobs once said, "I'm a big believer in boredom. . . . All the [technology] stuff is wonderful, but having nothing to do can be wonderful, too."

It is wonderful. And wonderfully rare. Boredom is now infrequent enough that the sight of someone doing nothing can be jarring. A friend of mine described a recent evening while he was lying in bed, staring at the ceiling and thinking. Just thinking. "My wife walked into the room, saw me, and asked if I was OK," he said. "She thought I'd had a stroke or something. It was too weird for her to see me just lying there not on my phone or laptop, with the TV turned off."

IT TAKES US ROUGHLY HALF AN HOUR TO REACH THE CLIFF. I'M SPENT. THESE 4 MILES felt like 14 on a typical mountain trail. I heave off my pack and dig into it for a half-frozen energy bar, which is about as easy to chew as a thick piece of cold leather. Donnie raises his binoculars and begins inspecting the mossy hillside. "I'm not seeing them," he says as he sweeps the top of the hill, the valley below it, and everything in between.

"Is that a herd over there?" asks William. He points to dots on a hill a mile or two to the northeast. Donnie drops the binoculars to squint. He brings them back to his eyes. "Shit," he says. "That has to be them." He dives into his bag and removes the spotting scope for a better view.

"Damn it. They must have picked up our scent as we moved along that ridge to get up to this cliff," he says. "Their scent is wicked. Just wicked. Man, can they move."

These caribou have a motor on them. They spend most of the day slowly grazing. But when they walk, it's a 12-mile-an-hour trot they can sustain for days. No Arctic predator will ever catch them in a sprint—caribou top out at 50 mph. And caribou biologists who track GPS data say the animals are constantly moving. They've reported collaring a caribou in one spot, the next day flying 50 miles to another spot, and finding the same caribou.

Even grizzlies can only kill a healthy caribou by ambush. Wolves work in a pack, converging on them from all angles. Both predators are unsuccessful more times than not. We have the same odds of catching this herd and that handsome bull as a sumo wrestler does winning the high jump at the next Olympic Games.

"So what do we do now?" I ask.

"It's quite possible there are more herds behind them," says Donnie. "So we'll just sit and glass from here and wait to see if any more come over the hill." It's one o'clock, 30 degrees, and the sun will set at 9:27.

So I found myself bored again. Again the game is waiting; waiting for caribou to move into view. Donnie once spent 42 ten-hour days waiting in the North Dakota woods for a single white-tailed deer.

The upside is that we've got a view unlike any I've seen. The tundra rolls on forever, stark and cold, and the sky is awash in grays. It's a muted beauty. I remove my cellphone from my pack, turn it on, and take a photo to share with family. It's a half-assed screen capture. A camera just can't reproduce this world's infinite vastness and haunting low-angle light.

"Feels nice not to be on that thing all the time, huh?" asks Donnie. I nod in agreement as I turn off the phone and repack it. "There are so few areas where you can't get service anymore," he says. "The only areas I find are when I'm hunting, and it's amazing."

"Do you ever get bored out here?" I ask.

Donnie keeps his eye in the spotting scope as he talks. "This might sound contrived. But, no, I don't get bored out here," he says. "There's so much to notice and learn. Like, did you hear the noise of that raven circling our camp this morning? It made this little 'boop boop' at us. They have such complex language. I've heard two or three raven vocalizations in just these few days that I've never heard before. Did you notice how there's always a raven nearby?"

The constant companionship of ravens hadn't struck me as odd. But Donnie is correct.

"They follow humans, bears, and wolves," he said. "They know we mean food. They'll pick our kill clean and even help us hunt. I've had ravens fly over me and squawk. Then they've flown to a nearby canyon or valley and squawked again. Sure enough, once I got to that location there was an animal. They're some of the smartest creatures on earth."

Donnie looks over at me and smiles. "OK, actually I do get bored sometimes," he says. "One time we got weathered into the tent for four days straight. We were so bored by day four that we just sat around reading labels looking for typos."

"We fuckin' found one, too!" adds William.

By 6 p.m. we've sat looking for no-show caribou for five straight hours. So we decide to call it a day. We have a few more hours of light. But locating a caribou, stalking it, killing it, and packing its meat back to camp would take far longer. That could put us in a dangerous position if an Arctic storm were to hit in the dark.

I sling my pack over my back, wishing I hadn't finished my lunch and snack bars by noon. I'm ravenous and we have a long walk ahead of us. "Well, boys," Donnie declares. "I think tomorrow we change course. We're not seeing enough caribou here."

This pleases me. A new mountainside to sit and do nothing on. A new landscape to view. New ground to inspect. A new slope to do push-ups on. Maybe a chance at caribou.

We begin the long trek back to camp. My mind feels like it's riding a different wavelength than the one it typically does back home. It's more a ripple than a riptide. Despite the cold, wind, and rough ground, my stress levels are nonexistent. Interesting new ideas are bubbling out of the ether. And I'm oddly appreciative—of the world around me but also of things back home. Like my wife. I can't wait to hear her sarcastic remark when I tell her how bored I've been. No one has perfected the art of giving me shit quite like she has, and it's never hit me how much that means to me.

I believe all these feelings have something to do with allowing my mind a moment of rest. Maybe when I get home, instead of thinking the oft-repeated "less phone," it might be more productive to think "more boredom."

12

20 MINUTES, 5 HOURS, 3 DAYS

BEFORE I ARRIVED in Alaska I came upon new research showing that, yeah, all our screen time is bad. But there's something else at play. What if our problem isn't just our screen time? What if all those hours we spend zoned into pixels aren't only adding something bad to our life but also removing us from something good?

We're nearing the end of our trek back to camp and following a game trail that runs along a rock- and moss-covered ridge. The trail is thin but well worn. It provides a welcome break from scrambling. Animals naturally take the path of least resistance to burn fewer calories. Which means that this trail is also an energy saver for us human animals.

"These game trails can be ten thousand years old," Donnie says. "In some areas, you'll find that the animals have all stepped in the same place, wearing down the exact same prints." The sun is preparing to drop into darkness. We're so far north that we lose four minutes of daylight each day. By Christmas this place will receive just two hours daily of good light.

As we curve along a steep ridge, the olive-green teepee comes into sight on a hill a mile away. And of course between us and the teepee is a herd of about 30 caribou. They're in a saddle set high between two hills.

"Standard," says Donnie. "We hike all day, get our ass kicked, and come back to find that caribou have been hanging out in camp." He pulls the binoculars to his eyes. William and I wait for a verdict.

This herd's proximity to camp means we could, despite how late it is, move in for a stalk. But I can't help feeling a kill this easy seems unsportsmanlike. I'm also aware that this notion is like playing God. If we were subsistence hunters, we would happily take the closest animal. Male or female, young or old. We'd just want dinner. The modern world has turned hunting, even the more morally conscious kind, into a reenactment of the past, and we therefore must insert ethics into the equation. Luckily we'll have no heady debates.

"There aren't old bulls in the group. Just young bulls, cows, and calves," Donnie says. "But they're stunning. Just stunning." I take the binoculars and focus on one calf. His long, lean muscles shift under his brown coat as he trots like a show pony. His breath fogs into the crisp air. "He's walking fancy, huh?" says Donnie.

William dumps his pack and changes the lens on his camera. "I'm going to get some footage." He hunches and tiptoes toward the herd. Donnie and I lie back on the slope and watch him close in. All is quiet.

William goes belly down about 400 yards from the animals and begins to crawl and film from the ground. After five minutes he starts moving in for a better angle.

Caribou move in herds because it's safer, not because they feel a particularly intimate bond with one another. They graze in open spaces. Their advantage is their speed, endurance, and eyesight. Having 30 pairs of eyes covering 360 degrees of land at different depths is safer than just one pair that covers a single direction. They'll see a bear or wolf coming from far enough away that they can simply stay out of range. Won't even stop eating.

William rises. One animal spooks and jukes away from him. This signals danger. The herd reacts, bobbing in sync like a flock of starlings. They gallop away from him across the tundra—directly toward Donnie and me.

The silence ends as they break 150 yards. The sound is at first a low rumble. But it's gaining decibels. The ground begins to vibrate. They're at 100 yards. Then 75. Then 50. The calf I saw is all skinny legs and lean body, galloping forward. Hooves smash the ground, kicking up moss and moisture. Then 40 yards, then 35.

I'm locked on them, completely in the here and now. We can hear their breathing, smell their coats, and see all the details of their ornate antlers.

One notices us and bobs. The group sweeps left, shaking the earth as they head uphill and summit a crest, their antlers black against a gold sunset.

Donnie and I are silent for a moment. Then I look at him. "Unbelievable, just unbelievable," he says. "Moments like that are why I come up here. Only by coming out here can you put yourself in a position to have wild moments and experiences like the one we just had." I'm also thinking it's unbelievable we didn't get trampled to death.

Those caribou shaking that patch of earth shook my soul. It was transcendent. Wild as a religious experience.

It's an experience we all should have. But probably not all at once in the same spot. Most of us today rarely experience the natural world. More than half of Americans don't go outside for any type of recreation at all. That includes the simple stuff like walking and jogging. The time we spend outdoors has declined over the past few decades, and American kids play outside 50 percent less than their parents did. Camping in the woods is down about 30 percent since 2006.

We shouldn't be surprised. Nature can be uncomfortable and unpredictable. In just a handful of days out here I've experienced savage weather, terrain that's put me flat on my face, haunting isolation, deafening quiet, and more. I never know what'll be around the next bend. It could be a storm rolling in, a steeper hill, a raging river, or an ill-tempered grizzly. The only thing I can predict is that I won't have cell service ever.

"If given a choice, human brains are going to say, 'Give me something that I can control or predict,'" said Dr. Judson Brewer, the Brown University Medical School psychiatrist. Humans evolved, he explained, to look to the future and track information that helped us survive. For example, knowing where our next meal was coming from. But now this fear of uncertainty oversteps its old boundaries, extending to many unknown circumstances. It's a form of comfort creep that traps us in the safety nets Donnie talks about.

Famed biologist E. O. Wilson developed a theory, called the biophilia hypothesis, which says we have an ingrained call to be in nature that's in competition with our evolutionary desire to control our environment. The thinking goes like this: We evolved in nature, and therefore have programmed within our genes a need to be in and connect with nature and living things. If we don't, we go a little haywire, as if we're missing a necessary nutrient for our body, mind, and sense of self.

After a handful of techless days trudging through Alaska, I was beginning to buy in to the theory. My brain was feeling less hunkered down in its typical foxhole—a state that I'd compare to a roadrunner on crystal meth, dementedly zooming from one thing to the next— and more like it belonged to a monk after a month at a meditation retreat. I just feel . . . better. Wilson put my feelings this way: "Nature holds the key to our aesthetic, intellectual, cognitive, and even spiritual satisfaction."

I'm not unique. Humans have long considered nature something of an organic Xanax. The Egyptians around 1550 BC, for example, had a complex network of "pleasure gardens" designed for the purpose of destressing. Cyrus the Great around 500 BC commissioned gardens for the crowded urban capital of Persia (present-day Iran) to improve his citizens' health and increase the sense of "calm" in his city.

And nearly every civilization since has had parks and gardens, places where humankind gets some sort of joy from spending time and effort toiling in the dirt just for the sake of looking at plants later on.

But science mostly considered these ideas and the biophilia hypothesis about as sound a discipline as astrology. Any benefits of nature, most thought, were just a by-product of what people in nature do—usually some kind of exercise, like hiking—rather than some sort of base-level intimate relationship we've developed with, like, peat moss. Then came the Japanese.

In the early 1980s, as Japan was becoming more urban and tech focused, the country's forest agency created a nature-based wellness program. They even coined a marketing term, *shinrin-yoku,* which translates to "forest bathing." The program essentially promoted sitting or walking in the woods and "taking in" nature.

The Japanese government told its citizens to improve their health by forest bathing. They even created parks across the country to do so. Japanese scientists then started to probe whether the tax-funded program had any positive impact. They've since published a flood of studies on shinrin-yoku—and pushed biophilia from hypothesis to hard science.

One of these Japanese studies found that people who spent about 15 minutes sitting in and then walking through nature experienced all kinds of drops in the measurements that doctors care about. Blood pressure readings, heart rates, and stress hormone levels all went down. In another study, people with the highest levels of stress felt a significant drop in anxiety, depression, and hostility after only two hours in the woods.

The Japanese scientists are so confident in the power of nature that they have bravely led out into the forest groups of people with bad hearts, kidneys, or immune systems. The people shuffled about and sat around and just generally "bathed" in the forest.

Each group showed improvements. The people with heart disease saw their blood pressure levels drop to those of a person a doctor might pass as healthy. Diabetics had blood sugar levels get close to a normal figure. The people with the weak immune systems started pumping out 150 percent more "natural killer" cells. These are the cells that, naturally, kill off the infections that are trying to kill you.

The Japanese have since done more than a hundred studies on shinrin-yoku. Their nearly-always-positive findings incited a global research trend.

The world is full of sick people, the number increasing rapidly the closer one gets to a sofa or soda fountain. Rates of chronic mental and physical diseases are skyrocketing across the world. But the way we deal with our sick isn't perfect. We treat symptoms not causes, pumping people full of expensive pills that come with astonishing side effects. Such as, I learned in a recent commercial for the anti-depressant medication Abilify, to take one example, "stroke in elderly people that can lead to death; neuroleptic malignant syndrome; un-controlled body movements; problems with your metabolism such as: high blood sugar and diabetes, increased fat levels in your blood, weight gain; unusual urges such as gambling, binge eating, compul-sive shopping and sexual urges; seizures; difficulty swallowing"; etc., etc., etc.

A walk in the woods is free. And to my knowledge it isn't linked to spastic, unplanned movements or urges to hurry down to the cor-ner store to spend your life savings on scratch-off lottery tickets and then bang the clerk who sold them to you. Perhaps most delightful of all, being treated by nature won't require you to haggle with some stonewalling health insurance company representative.

Across the globe there is now a network of legit nature research-ers studying all the ways the biophilia hypothesis might improve humans from head to toe. They're proving that the outdoors is one potent antidote to the modern human conditions of chronic disease and being overstressed, overstimulated, and overworked. They're also discovering how real people with jobs, kids, and commitments can easily work nature into their busy lives.

A few months before arriving in Alaska, I'd traveled to Boston to meet one of those legit nature scientists. She's got this big idea, a three-tiered approach to help overhaul our health and happiness. And she thinks it's possibly the best way to reclaim our zombie brains from the numbing effects of the modern world and leave us more joyful and our lives a little less insufferable.

THE FIELD OF NATURE SCIENTISTS TENDS TO BE RICH IN TREE HUGGERS WHO WERE good at school. A couple who have gained some notoriety, for example, live a lifestyle somewhere between scientist and 19th-century recluse. They don't own cellphones and live in off-the-grid homes with no Internet.

But I was in Boston to meet one who doesn't exactly fit that mold: Rachel Hopman. Wearing jeans, a T-shirt, and pink running shoes, she was sitting on a rock, hunched over her phone and swiping at its screen.

In my mind, it's one thing to be told by some about-to-retire earthy tech conspiracist that you need to go outside more and use your cellphone less. It's quite another to hear that message from Hopman, who was born in 1991, got her first cellphone at age 15, didn't grow up in an outdoorsy family, and loves a good iPhone binge. "I hadn't ever been camping until I was forced to in grad school," she told me. We'd started walking through the Arnold Arboretum, a Frederick Law Olmsted–designed 281-acre park roughly five miles southwest of the slip where the revolutionaries dumped tea into the Boston Harbor.

We know that time in nature is good. But Hopman's research is looking into exactly what doses we need across the days, months, and years for the optimal effects. And, critically, whether using our electronic devices alters those effects.

She noticed that she was still clutching her cellphone and smiled. "Today my phone notifies me any time I have more than sixty pickups or two hours and twenty minutes of screen time," she said. "That's more than some people expect, given what I research." She also admitted that she often hits that limit early in the day and says screw it and keeps on going. For her it's not about denying how amazing that little electronic rectangle is, it's about understanding what we lose when we use it.

We were walking past 100-foot-tall maple and spruce trees planted in the late 1800s, and she was telling me about her research. In 2016, she led a study that found something as painless as a 20-minute stroll through a city park, like the one we're in right now, can cause profound changes in the neurological structure of our brains. This leaves us feeling calmer and with sharper and more productive, creative minds. "But," she said, "we found that people who used their cellphone on the walk saw none of those benefits."

There's a little magic in 20 minutes. That was confirmed by Hopman's colleagues at the University of Michigan. They discovered that 20 minutes outside, three times a week, is the dose of nature that most efficiently dropped people's levels of the stress hormone cortisol. The catch to that study, of course, was that the participants couldn't take their phones outside with them.

In nature your brain enters a mode Hopman called "soft fascination." It's similar to unfocused mode—but with one key difference. "Instead of mind-wandering and lightly focusing inwardly, you're lightly focusing *outwardly* on the nature around you," she said. "You're taking in all these things in the outside world that are nice to look at. But they're not overwhelming. Your attention network is turned down, but you're aware of the outside world."

If this brand of present-moment awareness sounds a lot like something yogis chase, that's because it basically is. Brain scans show that soft fascination is a lot like meditation. Hopman described it as a mindfulness-like state that restores and builds the resources we need to think, create, process information, and execute tasks. It's mindfulness without the meditation. A short, daily nature walk is a great option for people who aren't keen on sitting and focusing on their breath. Of course, a walk in the woods only becomes mind medicine so long as the phone is away and also not beaming information into our ears.

In today's economy, where people can't detach from work emails, nearly a quarter to half of all employees say they're burned out. Nature may be the best recovery tool for the condition, said Hopman. Say mind-wandering at home is akin to taking a hot bath after a tough workout. Mind-wandering in nature might be like taking that hot bath, then drinking a protein shake and getting a massage.

"Every now and then after I give a talk a person will come up to me and ask, 'How do you expect people who work to spend time outside? It's just, like, one more thing on the long list of things that scientists tell me I have to do for my health,'" Hopman said as we veered off the paved path onto a dirt trail that cut through a woody marsh. "I tell those people it doesn't have to be complicated. Just passing through a park or by some trees on a walk to a coffee shop has benefits. Almost immediately when people are in nature or even see nature they report feeling better and their behavior changes."

As the University of Michigan scientists found, the ideal quick dose is 20 minutes, three times a week, of this, let's call it, "urban nature" that's found in cities, suburbs, and towns. But we can be even lazier than that and still experience benefits. Hopman began firing off facts about just how little nature it takes to be better off.

"Having plants in your office can increase your productivity," she said. One study—conducted across multiple offices with hundreds of workers—found the boost was about 15 percent more work completed. The workers also said they liked their jobs more.

"There's other research that shows even having a view of nature out of a hospital window helps people recover quicker," said Hopman. That one, published in *Science* in 1984, also found that the patients with window views had fewer complications, complained less, and didn't need to pop as many pain pills.

"Even taking a route to work where you see more green is beneficial," she said. The study gathered surveys of thousands of workers from cities both minuscule and massive. It found that people who passed the most green space commuting to work had better mental health.

"And people who live near green spaces are less at risk of all kinds of diseases," she said. A review investigated 143 studies on the topic. It showed those people were less likely to have heart attacks, strokes, asthma, and diabetes, and were also more likely to survive if they had cancer.

This is why it's important to stop thinking that nature, as Yale professor Steven Kellert said, is "out there, somewhere else." Like it's a place that exists only in *National Geographic* or on voyages to Alaska. Nature is often right outside your window, in your backyard, lining your block, and in that park down the street.

"People are busy," said Hopman. "I get it." Some days you'll have a pile of work. A walk through a park seems unfeasible. Any time away from the grind feels like too much time away from the grind. "I tell busy people about the productivity and creativity benefits of nature," she said. Think of that short walk outside like a high-return investment in yourself. Those 20 minutes in the park may cause you to pump out, say, 20 widgets instead of the 18 you would have done had you tried to power through the day in burnout mode. And perhaps those widgets would be more creatively designed.

Twenty minutes, three times a week, is great. But it's at the bottom of what some nature scientists have dubbed "the nature pyramid." Think of this like the food pyramid. Except that instead of recommending that you eat this many servings of vegetables and this many of meat, it recommends the ideal amounts of time you should spend in nature and how often. Tomorrow we'd take a step up the pyramid.

Hopman also promised to reveal to me what her research found about the pinnacle of the pyramid, that highest point, where our minds get completely blown, undergoing a sort of hard reset.

THE NEXT DAY I MET HER AT BLUE HILLS RESERVATION, A 7,000-ACRE STATE PARK south of Boston. We'd been ascending a rocky, mossy trail for the last hour and were just about to top out. Think of this type of nature as "country nature." It's wilder than the landscaped, manicured stuff you'll find in a park or your backyard. But it's not so far removed. You can get there by a quick car or bus ride.

"Any time in nature is beneficial," said Hopman as we reached the crest of the trail. "But spending more time in wilder spaces does seem to give you more benefits." Time in this semiwild stuff comprises level two of the nature pyramid. Research, in part thanks to Finland, says we should spend a total of about five hours in it a month.

About 95 percent of Finns spend time outdoors. The country realized the Japanese were onto something and did a bit of forest bathing research of their own. The Finnish government surveyed thousands of their citizens. It wanted to know what dose of nature seemed to do the most good.

Most people in the survey said they felt best on about five hours a month. With that amount of time they were more likely to avoid depression (it's easy to get depressed in the long, dark winters of Finland) and be happier in their everyday lives.

The government then followed up on that survey with a legitimate study contrasting one group of people in a city center, another in a city park, and another in a country park. They discovered that the groups who spent time in the urban and wilder parks felt more tranquil than the people dropped off in the city. No shocker there. Except the people in the wilder country space had an edge over the city park people. They felt even more relaxed and restored. The takeaway: The wilder the nature, the better.

Hopman and I paused at the hill's rocky top with trees at our back and sides. Before us was a view of the Atlantic Ocean, miles and miles away. The scene was nice enough that I stopped questioning Hopman for a moment. We stood there taking it in. "See, you definitely couldn't get this from a city park," she said.

There could be a lot of reasons why nature—wilder spaces in particular—has these effects on the mind and body. It could be that in nature you are engulfed in fractals, complex patterns that repeat over and over in different sizes and scales and make up the design of the universe. Think trees (big branch to smaller branch to smaller branch and so on), river systems (little river to bigger river to bigger river and so on), mountain ranges, clouds, seashells. "Cities don't have fractals," said Hopman. "Think of a typical building. It's usually flat, with right angles. It's painted some dull color." Fractals are organized chaos, which our brains apparently dig. In fact, scientists at the University of Oregon discovered that Jackson Pollock's booze- and jazz-induced paintings are made up of fractals. This may explain why they speak to humans at a core level.

Or it could be the smells of nature. Or the sunlight. Or just the fact that you're getting out of the stress of your home or office. "It's probably a mix of a lot of things," said Hopman. Things that cities, with their frenetic pace, right angles, loud noise, rotten smells, pinging phones, and to-do lists don't offer.

I did the math as we stared at the water. "So five hours. That's, like, maybe one or two hikes, picnics, fishing trips, or mountain bike rides a month?" I said.

"Yep, exactly," Hopman replied. Which explains why I'd felt so chilled out training for the Alaskan voyage. Those weekly hikes weren't just prepping my body. They were also medicating my mind.

MY TRIP TO ALASKA IS AT THE TOP OF THE NATURE PYRAMID. AND IT TURNS OUT THAT what's enchanted my brain there is a certifiable scientific phenomenon. It even has a catchy name, "the three-day effect." To experience this level requires "backcountry nature." A trip into the wild places that begin where dirt roads end. Places characterized by spotty cell reception, wild animals, and a lack of bathrooms and other humans.

I'm telling Donnie about my time with Hopman and this effect as we arrive in camp. The teepee is a big triangle, black against the orange sky. We heave off our packs and dump them on the ground.

"This three-day effect she studies basically says that a few days in nature change your mind for the better," I tell him as I rummage my pack for my down jacket. "More time in nature seems to make people calmer. More at peace, more present, more appreciative. Happier. That kind of stuff. And the effect seems to last after you leave."

"Do you think that's why I come out here?" he asks.

"Do *you* think that's why you come out here?" I respond.

"Hmmm," he says. "Well, I know the longer you're here, the better. That's for sure. More time benefits you more as a human. I've seen it in me and I've seen it in others. I feel more at peace and start to become part of the land, part of the ecosystem. I love the sunrises and sunsets. I love seeing the animals. What we just saw with those caribou. That fills my mind and soul. I'll think about those caribou ten, twenty, thirty years from now."

The wind has settled, and the herd has climbed to the safety of a ridge. We stand and eye them, black specks on the horizon.

Donnie continues. "I'm always so incredibly inspired when I'm here and when I get back home," he says. He's kneeling now, rifling through his pack. He pulls out his own down jacket. A chill is settling in now that we've stopped moving. "I agree that the feeling lasts for a while, too."

Research into the three-day effect was spurred on by Ken Sanders, a Salt Lake City icon, rare-book dealer, and longtime friend of environmental writer and general badass Edward Abbey.

"From decades of river rafting going back to the 1980s, I've long been aware of the metamorphosis or transformation that occurs on day three of wilderness trips," Sanders told me from his bookstore in downtown Salt Lake City.

Sanders happened to mention his personal experiences with the three-day effect to David Strayer. Strayer is a hardcore nature junkie, a University of Utah neuroscientist, and the world's foremost expert on how cellphones affect attention and the brain.

For Strayer the phrase was less a tagline and more a lightbulb firing on.

In Stayer's many years of backpacking through the red rock canyons of southern Utah, he'd experienced the buzz himself. That calm, altered spectrum of thinking that seems to enhance perception and peacefulness and dial back time and space. He'd even had conversations with friends and other academics who'd experienced the same. But he'd never heard a timeline stamped on it. He wondered if the three-day effect was something he could study.

Strayer gave it a try in 2012. He and his team talked their way onto a handful of Outward Bound backpacking trips. The rule: No cellphones in the wilderness.

Half of the Outward Bound students the morning before their trip took the RAT for creativity (the test where three words are thrown out and we have to figure out their common denominator). The other half took the test after their third techless day in the backcountry. The people who were tested after the wilderness trip scored 50 percent better. Strayer thought he might see an improvement by day three. But 50 percent? That's no fluke.

It was enough to establish the three-day effect as a concept worth chasing. The research has been building since. Another study found that people who spent a handful of days paddling the water of the Minnesota backcountry scored much higher on the RAT compared to people who took it indoors. Another piece of research discovered that vets who spent six days on a backcountry trip saw their stress symptoms plummet.

We now know that the three-day effect doesn't wash off once we're back home. Scientists at UC Berkeley found that US military vets who spent four days rafting in southern Utah were still feeling the effects a week later. Their PTSD symptoms and stress levels were down 29 and 21 percent, respectively. Their relationships, happiness, and general satisfaction with their lives were all improved as well.

John Muir in 1901 put it this way: "Nerve-shaken, over-civilized people are beginning to find out that going to the mountains is going home; that wilderness is a necessity; and that mountain parks and reservations are useful not only as fountains of timber and irrigating rivers, but as fountains of life."

Three or more days in the wild is like a meditation retreat. Except talking is allowed and the experience is free of costs and gurus.

The rewilding of our body and brain usually goes something like this: On the first day stress and health markers improve, but we are still adjusting to the discomfort of nature. We're thinking about how it sucks to be cold, missing our phone, and still focusing on the anxieties we left behind—what's happening at work and whether we closed the garage door. By day two our mind is settling and aware-ness is heightening. We're caring less about what we left behind and are beginning to notice the sights, smells, and sounds around us. Then day three hits.

Now our senses are completely dialed in and we can reach a fully meditative mode of feeling connected to nature. The discomfort isn't so bad. It has, in fact, shifted to a welcome sensation that signals a calmness and feeling of life satisfaction.

Which brings us back to Strayer and Hopman. Strayer started a class that delves into the psychological benefits of nature. Hopman was his graduate student at the time. For the course's capstone, the two would take the students camping for four days into one of the most remote spots in the Lower 48: Sand Island Campground out-side Bluff, Utah.

The kids were allowed to bring their cellphones. But, sadistically, Hopman didn't mention that there's no service within miles of the campsite. So the 18- to 22-year-olds would arrive, try to post out-door photos to Instagram, be stonewalled, and then go through the five stages of receptionless grief. There was denial, where they'd walk around, arm in the air, trying to get service; anger, where they'd curse their service provider and toss their phone into the tent; bargaining, where they'd consider hiking to a nearby peak to perhaps get service; depression, where they'd long deeply to post that status update; and, finally, acceptance, where they'd realize, hey, I may actually survive and this phoneless nature stuff isn't so bad after all.

Somewhere between denial, anger, and bargaining, on day one, Hopman would have strapped complicated brain-wave measuring devices onto the skulls of the students. Three days later, once the students had hit acceptance, she'd retest them.

The students' day-one brain waves were beta waves. These are frenetic, type-A, go-go-go waves. But by day three they'd be riding what are called alpha and theta waves. These are the same waves found in experienced meditators and people who have lapsed into an effortless flow state. These rare waves reset your thinking, revive your brain, tame burnout, and just make you feel better.

"You don't really see the good alpha and theta waves appear in the short excursions outside," said Hopman. "That's why taking a backcountry trip each year is so important." We in the modern world are riding high, violent beta brain waves more often than any humans in history, and the message is clear: Time in nature is a hell of a way to calm the turbulent sea inside our minds.

12 PLACES

THE MORNINGS ARE special. It's now 7:45 a.m. on day six. I wake inside my straitjacket-like mummy sleeping bag that's laid atop an inch-thick blow-up sleeping pad. My head is resting on a pillow of smelly, wadded-up clothes. The teepee is below freezing. Despite these accommodations, I've slept nine to ten perfect hours each night.

I'm working hard every day. But my stellar sleep pattern also has to do with the darkness and silence, according to Chris Winter, MD, a neurologist and sleep researcher. A third of Americans regularly sleep less than seven hours a night. Winter says most modern sleep problems are caused by the fact that we are rarely in adequate darkness and silence—two nighttime qualities that humans evolved to sleep in. The fact that we rarely physically exhaust ourselves also factors in.

I quietly exit my bag, slip on my camp shoes, and tiptoe to the entrance of the teepee. A tiny snowstorm of frost falls from its walls as I pull its door zipper. The mossy ground is frozen. It crunches beneath my feet as I walk to the top of the mesa above camp.

The snowy peaks of the Brooks Range mountains are illuminating to the north, and the eastern sky is cantaloupe and pocked with gray and shining white clouds. There is no wind.

I hear only the muted churn of a distant river and my own breathing. I stand there for a long time, listening to the nothing. Eventually

I pick up another sound. It's my heart beating. It begins to thump in my ears. Then I can hear the inner workings of my lungs. This is, undoubtedly, the most quiet I've ever experienced.

I could stand here all day and this quiet would remain unaltered by commuters, airplanes, construction, the hum of mechanical devices, and all the other noises of the modern world.

Then I pick up another sound. It begins gently, but it's gaining volume and coming in fast. It's a low whooshing. I turn to find it. Nothing. It's getting louder. *Whoosh, whoosh, whoosh.* I look up. *WHOOSH, WHOOSH, WHOOSH.* A raven is flying directly overhead, her coal wings able to, in all that silence, produce a sound like an Apache helicopter.

It's not that the wings of the birds in our cities and towns aren't making this sound. Or that the rivers, winds, and wildlife everywhere don't emit their own sort of music. It's just that so much of their sound is drowned out by all the noise we humans are making. The silence of the natural world is increasingly hard to find.

THE THING ABOUT SILENCE IS THAT IT'S NOWHERE. THAT'S WHAT THEORETICAL physics tells us, anyway. Even the quietest places are inundated with white noise, the sound that electromagnetic waves make as they travel through space. White noise can exist even in the vacuum of outer space. You may not hear it, but white noise is engulfing you at this moment.

In Alaska I'm swimming through white noise. And also the sound of the wind cutting over the tundra tussocks, frozen ground crunching underfoot, distant rivers rolling, ravens whooshing their wings and speaking their ever-evolving dialect, the inner workings of my body, and more.

It's a relief to be away from the noise I'm used to. Before I got up here, one morning I went out to my back patio and set a timer for one minute. Then I sat on a wooden recliner, kicked up my legs, and listened. I noticed birdsong and wind flowing through the palms. Then I heard cars speeding, a car door slamming, a car horn blaring, a plane roaring, electricity humming, and my dog whining that it was breakfast time and I should finish this silly experiment and feed him. Stop and listen. The noise is everywhere.

Over time, explains Harvard anthropologist Daniel Lieberman, humans have removed from our environment many sensory inputs. For example, we feel fewer temperature swings. We wear shoes, so our feet feel less. We smell less, because we rarely have to smell food to determine if it's safe (and what we do smell is generally pleasant, like hand soap), etc. But he said this rule does not hold for our hearing.

Humans have increased the world's loudness fourfold. Scientists at the University of Michigan say that more than 100 million Americans live with noise levels louder than what you'd hear standing next to a working washing machine or dishwasher. That's 70 decibels.

We have in fact become so used to living with noise that most of us now find comfort in constant blare, according to a scientist in Australia. The researcher had hundreds of students spend a little time in the quiet and write about their experiences. Nearly every student said the silence made them uneasy. "The lack of noise made me uncomfortable, it actually seemed foreboding," wrote one student. "Perhaps because media consistently surrounds us today, we have a fear of peace and quiet," wrote another.

Another survey found that Americans increasingly see the TV not as an entertainment device but as a companion. More than half of us keep the TV on while we work, cook, and do chores because we feel uncomfortable in silence. Silence-induced discomfort is a new, learned behavior, those Australian scientists think.

Humans evolved in a soundscape like the one I'm experiencing in the Arctic. Our days were quiet, and any loud noises usually signaled trouble. Like a roar from a predator or an enemy, the booms of a violent storm, or the crash of a rockslide.

Our brains are wired to think loud = danger. We react by releasing adrenaline and cortisol, stress hormones that kick on the fight-or-flight response. Our doses of noise-induced stress hormones used to be infrequent but lifesaving.

Today's jarring background noises spur the same fight-or-flight response. But the difference is that these noises are nearly constant. This makes our hormones behave like a slow-dripping water torture, and the constant noise is more than enough to stress us out, according to the CDC. Marinating in stress has consequences.

In fact, the world's number-one killer, heart disease, isn't just a consequence of too much couch and carbs. The World Health Organization found that the constant stream of decibels we live in is, quite literally, taking years off our lives. Too much noise was responsible for nearly 2,000 heart attack deaths in Europe. This is because stress increases can lead to heart disease.

Other research shows antianxiety medication use rises a relative 28 percent for every 10-decibel increase a neighborhood experiences, and people who live near loud roads are 25 percent more likely to be depressed. Other studies show that background noise also impairs our attention, memory, learning, and interactions with others.

And the thing is, we don't even realize the noise is dragging us down, according to scientists at Cornell. They had two groups of office workers complete a project. One group worked in a quiet office. The other worked in an open-concept office. That open-concept office was 50 percent louder, thanks to the annoyances of ringing phones, the clacks of fingers hitting keyboards, people talking about bottom lines, etc.

The workers in the loud office said they didn't feel any more stressed than the workers in the quiet office. But the data said otherwise. Their bodies pumped out significantly more of the stress hormone adrenaline and they completed less work. They were also less motivated to work.

Silence is worth seeking, even if it's uncomfortable at first. Where can we find unadulterated natural silence? An acoustic ecologist (real job, apparently) named Gordon Hempton traveled the country in search of silence. He now believes that there are only 12 places in the Lower 48 where we can sit for 15 minutes and not hear a single noise created by humans. No droning planes, trains, automobiles. No blaring TVs, cellphones, or radios. Just natural soundscape. Some of these 12 places are spots in Minnesota's Boundary Waters Canoe Area Wilderness, Hawaii's Haleakala National Park, and Washington's Hoh River Valley.

North America's other consistently quiet places are way up north, where I am: Alaska, the Arctic, Yukon, Northwest Territories, etc.

But just because silence is hard to find doesn't mean we shouldn't seek it. Because, I'd learn from an aging sound nerd, incredible things happen the closer people come to silence. And we don't necessarily have to go to points north to find it.

THE CLOSEST WE CAN GET TO SILENCE IS IN A DRAB GRAY BUILDING ACROSS FROM a city park and an old liquor store on 2709 East Twenty-fifth Street in Minneapolis, Minnesota.

Orfield Laboratories, run by Steven Orfield, is a small Twin Cities business that leverages the power of perception to help companies build better products. Harley-Davidson, for example, once hired Orfield to calculate the exact engine tone and decibel level that would give riders the impression that its motorcycles are powerful.

The guy's lab has a long history of sound. It was the world's first digital recording studio. Prince got his start at Orfield Labs. Bob Dylan even recorded half of *Blood on the Tracks* there. But one day in 1992, Orfield received a curious call that would make his lab known for something else. The guy on the other end of the landline was a fellow audio nerd who had a hot tip.

"He told me that the appliance maker Sunbeam corporation was closing their US research lab," Orfield told me. "The CEO had told the research employees, 'Sell anything you can get rid of to make us money.' So Sunbeam was selling an anechoic chamber and all the equipment that comes with it."

An anechoic chamber is a completely silent room. The inside contains a platform for standing and the walls, ceiling, and floor are layered in sound-killing foam cones. Orfield, however, would be facing some stiff competition. "Motorola and IBM also wanted to buy the chamber," he said.

So here was Orfield, a Minnesota audio dork, with his Minnesota accent, naive friendliness, and limited budget. And he was bidding against two of the largest tech corporations in the world. But Orfield had something those two mega-companies didn't: no bureaucracy and a checkbook sitting right there on his desk.

"I guess Sunbeam's CEO had said the company had to sell all the equipment in two weeks," said Orfield. "IBM and Motorola couldn't move that fast. So I bought the chamber. I didn't even have a building to put it in."

Three semitrucks loaded with the massive room of silence arrived a week later at a Minneapolis storage facility. The room sat there for seven years, until Orfield had the money to add a wing onto his lab.

When people first enter the chamber, they feel uncomfortable with the silence, said Orfield. The lack of noise is a sensation unlike any they've had. "But then people start to calm down," he said. And they become progressively more pacified, during which their perception of sound recalibrates and begins to settle. Then they reach the 30-minute mark.

"That's when people start to hear the sounds their ears make," said Orfield. "Then they hear their heart beat, and the joints in their arms and legs moving. Some people hear the flowing in their lungs and the blood from their carotid artery spreading into their brain. People go into the chamber thinking they're going to hear silence. But what they get is the sound of themselves." The thing about silence is that it's nowhere, indeed.

But this recalibration, this heightening of our lowest levels of perception, leaves us calmer and less anxious. It scrubs the brain of the stress-inducing noise we live in, according to Orfield. "People go into the chamber and come out saying things like 'My brain hasn't felt this good in years,'" he said. "We had someone who was on an aircraft carrier in the Middle East. He could still hear the planes taking off. He went into the chamber and afterward the noise was gone. It had reset his hearing back to zero." Orfield's anechoic chamber has since been named the quietest place on earth by Guinness World Records.

Extreme quiet is a promising treatment for people who've gone through trauma, particularly vets suffering from PTSD. When he retires, Orfield plans to flip his lab into a nonprofit that will be used for therapy and research.

It's probably not feasible to lounge in Orfield's lab. But just leaving the sounds of the city has huge benefits. "You take someone who's in a city and put them in the sounds of a park and they immediately become calmer," said Orfield.

Hearing the natural sounds we evolved in seems to strike a calming note within us. Scientists in the UK, for example, found that people who listened to nature sounds like water and wind reduced their stress levels significantly more than those who listened to artificial noises.

We also know that seeking the everyday silence that comes from shutting off devices can benefit our brain and body. Two hours of the type of quiet we can find at home (perhaps with earplugs in or noise-canceling headphones on, if you live in a city) was shown to lead to the production of more cells in an area of the brain that fights depression. The study showed that at-home silence was more calming than listening to Mozart. Other research found that two minutes of silence led to the bigger drops in measures of relaxation like blood pressure and heart and breathing rate compared to a handful of other relaxation techniques. Yes, silence is more relaxing than most of the "relaxing" products marketers try to sell us.

I HEAR MY JOINTS CREAK AS I TURN AND BEGIN THE WALK BACK TO THE TEEPEE. THE sun is rising low and slow on the horizon.

I unzip the teepee to find William mummified in his bag and Donnie sitting on the edge of his pad. He's boiling water on our back-packing stove. Steam rises from the pot and exits his mouth as he asks, "What were you doing out there?"

"Just listening," I say. "Listening to the silence."

"It's wild, right?" he says. "The silence alone is worth the price of admission."

PART THREE

Feel hunger.

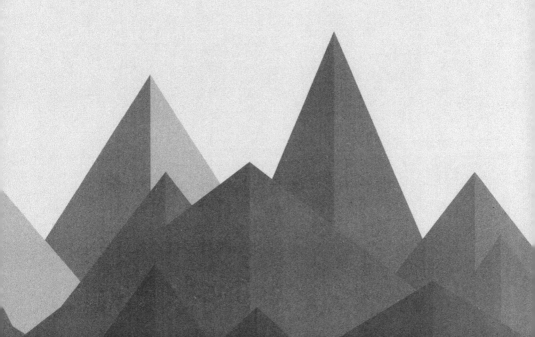

14

-4,000 CALORIES

"WE'RE GETTING INTO the lean times, boys!" William declares as he cinches his belt, the waistband of his pants bunching as the leather strap slides through its brass buckle.

The weather turned snowy last night. Three inches of powder now coat the ground.

After our unsuccessful stalk, we hung around the ridge at camp for a couple of days, thinking the animals would come to us. Nothing. The next few days we hiked miles in the opposite direction, thinking those valleys might reveal migrating herds. Nothing.

But a couple of days ago, at a location far from camp, we watched a mother caribou and her young calf evade a pack of wolves, eventually trotting just a hundred yards from us. It was a sign. A sign that caribou might be on their way. Today we'll return to that spot, but we're taking our time getting there.

After repeated river crossings yesterday, every boot in camp this morning was frozen solid. Putting them on was a ten-minute process. I'd jam my foot as far into the icy block as I could. Then I'd wait until my foot thawed that section of boot enough for me to press another few centimeters deeper. So on and so forth. Time, pressure, and a little heat; the same forces that build mountains and forge diamonds.

When I stepped out of the teepee my frozen boots caused me to walk like some Wild West cowboy, all swinging hips and knees.

"We're going to eat like kings if today goes well," Donnie says as we take the first steps out of camp. "Mark my word, boys. We'll eat steaks and double Mountain House dinners." The sun is rising and a thick frost covers everything. Rays bounce off billions of frozen crystals, rendering the land shimmering white.

"Do you think you could finish a steak and two Mountain House dinners?" I ask in a skeptical tone.

"Oh, fuck yeah I could," says William. "After we got stranded in the Yukon without food for four days, we immediately went to this Chinese restaurant and ordered two hundred dollars' worth of these appetizer platters that had all kinds of fried shit like wontons, egg rolls, chicken wings, pot stickers, crab Rangoon. We fuckin' destroyed it all. De. Stroyed. It."

Group conversations increasingly focus on food. Talk of how we're running low and will have to ration. Talk of caribou steaks. Talk of our first stop after coming out of the Arctic: "Moose's Tooth Pub and Pizzeria for the best pizza in Alaska," Donnie declares. "And we're going to sit down, order the entire menu, and just *crush* pizza."

We're facing what I guess I'd call a hunger-induced food obsession. We're now so damn ravenous that our mental energies revolve around food and how we can get it, the state increasing the further we dig ourselves into this hunger hole.

And digging we are. Yesterday we each consumed about 2,000 calories. That's granola for breakfast, a couple of energy bars for lunch, and a Mountain House dinner. We need three times that to stay healthy. A day out here burns roughly 6,000 calories, putting us 4,000 in the hole each day, our total deficit falling further into the red the more days we go without caribou.

At camp last night we flocked around the stove like a conspiracy of ravens on a kill, together waiting for the water to boil so we could pour it into our dinner bags.

"It's funny," Donnie said as we stood around, ravaging our meals. "We're out here searching for the purest, most delicious protein on the planet, and we're rifling down this ultraprocessed shit."

Lasagna with meat sauce was my ultraprocessed bag of choice. The freeze-dried ground beef hydrates into deer-scat-like pellets, while the cheese develops the consistency of spackling paste that sticks to my plastic camping spoon and must later be scraped off with a fingernail.

But the forced, core-deep hunger of this hunt has a way of taking this dish to something edible. Tasty, even.

"After a really rough sheep hunt in Tok, I came out of the woods starving, but all the local businesses were closed. I was forced to spend a shitty night in this old, mouse-filled abandoned Conex box," Donnie told us as we ate. "I found this pack of saltines that'd been in there for years. I thought about it for about five seconds then ate them all. They were unbelievably good in that moment." Hunger, apparently, is the best sauce.

I reached the bottom of my dinner bag far too soon and still felt hollow as I returned to the teepee.

There I crouched and took stock of my protein bars, counting and recounting them like you might ammunition before a firefight. My pace of eating two a day is unsustainable. So I placed one bar deep in my bag for the following day. I didn't want it accessible, where I might be tempted to eat it early. I then lay there, anticipating breakfast in ten hours. I've gone to bed increasingly hungry each night. The hunger comes in waves—cresting and breaking throughout the day. But at night, when I have nothing to do but think about food, the hunger hits hard, pushing deep into my stomach and throat.

BEFORE THIS ALASKA TRIP, I DON'T THINK I'D ACTUALLY EVER EXPERIENCED A PROB-lem with hunger. Food's always been available and I usually ate it because it was time for breakfast, lunch, or dinner. Or because I was stressed or bored. Or because it was just . . . there. The Japanese call this *kuchisabishii,* which literally means "lonely mouth" and describes our constant mindless eating. I couldn't recall the last time I experienced stomach-deep hunger lasting more than a day.

Food insecurity, defined as not having reliable access to food, is a problem in America—particularly among children, who must rely on others to eat. But the much larger problem seems to be an epidemic of too many of us never feeling hungry. As I noted in chapter 3, more than 70 percent of the country is overweight or obese—a figure that's projected to be 86.2 percent by 2030—and obesity takes an average of 5 to 20 years off a person's life, according to a study in *JAMA.*

Eating for reasons beyond hunger combined with effortless access to cheap, calorie-rich ultraprocessed food is creating a country that looks a lot like the passengers on the ship in *Wall-E*—bloated and lethargic.

Yet the solutions we're given to this problem are messy and convoluted. I've regularly written and reported on nutrition research and diet culture for years, and even as somewhat of an expert in this field, I've found it increasingly hard to know what information is actually useful. This confusion is due in no small amount to the lobbying, research, and marketing money spent by Big Nutrition.

One month a scientific study will show that carbs—or fat, or meat, or sugar—are good for us. The next month some other study will suggest that no, no, they are actually killing us. One year a cleverly named diet will rise in popularity by claiming it has the Secret that no one is telling us. The next some other will take the lead by preaching that every diet that came before it is all wrong, and that *it* is actually the holder of some coveted fitness and fat-loss formula.

And the so-called experts don't exactly clarify things. Nutrition scientists are separated into warring factions and can be so dug into their ideological corners that it's hard to figure out who's right. One scientific misconduct watchdog I interviewed described the world of nutrition science as "like the Hatfields and McCoys. Except there are maybe five families. And if they don't hate each other, they're great actors."

And what these scientists often study is usually too vague, too down-the-rabbit-hole, or too impractical for a real person with real problems. Researchers, after all, don't help people lose weight in a real-world setting.

Nutritionists, of course, work with real people. But many don't deeply grasp the biological underpinnings and are too busy regurgitating fad diet pseudoscience: "low-fat diet: fat is the problem, don't eat fat"; "keto diet: carbs are the problem, don't eat carbs"; "paleo diet: foods outside of the Paleolithic era are the problem, so eat only foods a caveman would eat"; "carnivore diet: foods that aren't meat are the problem, so eat meat only"; "Mediterranean, Okinawan, and Nordic diets: foods from elsewhere are the problem, so only eat foods from the Mediterranean, Okinawa, or Scandinavia."

And these nutritionists often suggest that if we don't follow their restrictive and complicated meal plan then we are lazy or lacking willpower, or both (as if people are alien robots who have no clue what's healthy and unhealthy and only need an impractical list of magical foods to succeed).

To top it all off, scientists and nutritionists alike often receive funding from different industries (which they often don't disclose). This, research shows time and time again, leads to studies and recommendations that favor the industry (such as meat, dairy, grain) that cut the check.

And here's the thing: Humans figured out that the amount of food we eat has something to do with our body size about 2,300 years ago. We could have stopped the research then. But we've since spent billions proving and re-proving that the ancients had it right: Eating less of something—carbs, fat, sugar, etc.—causes us to . . . eat less and therefore lose weight.

And we also know now that all diets work until they don't. Which is, according to one large survey in the UK, an average of 5 weeks,

2 days, and 43 minutes in. That's when we give up and slowly slide back into our previous state.

Why? This is when the discomfort sets in. People usually fail after a handful of weeks because their bodies fight to bring them back to their starting point. When your body fat drops enough, your brain responds by making you hungrier while at the same time decreasing how satisfying your meals are. A team at the NIH recently found that for every two pounds a person loses, for example, their brain unconsciously ramps up their hunger and causes them to eat about 100 more calories. Had our bodies not developed these defense mechanisms, we likely wouldn't have survived the crucible of evolution.

This is why fad diets aren't solving the nation's weight problem. It's not information and advice we lack (after all, fad diets work when followed consistently over the long run). It's our inability to persist against the discomfort of hunger—a necessary state for weight loss. Just 3 percent of the people who lose weight in a given year manage to keep it off. Their secret isn't some special food or exercise no one else has. It's their ability to get comfortable with discomfort.

A handful of years ago, I stumbled upon an unexpected new voice in the nutrition space. I first heard about him like you might an underground fight club, and he was described to me as "the *outsider* insider." I was reporting on a complex health story and had struck out on finding a satisfying answer to a question about the health effects of processed food.

After too many futile phone calls, a PhD source passed along his name, Trevor Kashey, and a nondescript email address. "This kid will probably give you a good answer," she said. "He understands the science at a very deep level, but he stands outside of it. He hasn't been incorporated into the machine in the way a lot of nutrition experts are, who can't see out of it."

An enlightened outsider. Someone who, as the source put it, "can go down the rabbit hole, as crazy deep as you could ever go but is able to capture things extremely succinctly, beautifully, and elegantly and who really knows exactly what to prioritize for real people. And is also accepting of any diet or way of eating you want to try." No ideological bias. No industry funding.

Just, I'd learn, a recognition that discomfort is inherent to physical change—whether losing weight or fueling an athletic goal—and innovative guidance to help people win the inner game of hunger.

And the approach was working. Kashey's clients had lost—and kept off—a collective 245,897 pounds and worked with him for an average of two years. They left only because he'd given them the tools to own their discomfort and permanently rewire their eating habits.

I emailed him a request to chat and received a 3:00 a.m. response saying that the discussion would be better over webcam. But, he explained, he was currently in Azerbaijan working with that nation's Olympic combat sports team, so we'd need to find a time that worked for both of our zones.

The video came through overly pixelated, and the man on the other end did not exactly fit the monotone, bespectacled, white-lab-coat nutritionists I was used to. He was in his early 20s, mohawked, and bearded. "Jesus! It's great to hear American English," he said. "And how can I be of service to you today, good sir?"

I started by asking the same softball question I'd asked every source I'd interviewed for the story: "Why is processed food so unhealthy?"

He looked at me like you might a person who believes the world is flat. "Is it, though?" he asked, and paused.

I raised my eyebrows and said, "Ummmm . . . ," as I figured out how to respond.

"Let's back up," he continued. "Do you know *why* we process food?"

"Well . . . ," I said. "Because it . . ." I trailed off. Apparently I did not.

"There are basically three reasons," he said. "The number-one priority is to keep a food safe, the next is to transport it to areas that can't cultivate their own food, and the third is to maintain the texture, flavor, and mineral and vitamin content in storage. For example, meat starts to spoil if we don't immediately cool it, cook it, or salt it, which are all forms of processing. Vegetables and grains are often treated with pesticides, cleaned, cut, flash frozen, blanched, or canned to maintain their freshness. So if you think processed food is bad, well, then, tell me what you think would happen if we didn't process food?"

I sat there, eyes squinted, processing the information as he continued.

"Processing food is literally the cornerstone of human civilization. Hunting, foraging, and farming only go so far. It's *keeping* food that's hard. It used to be that you could only grow food a few months out of the year and then you'd just pray to whatever deities you worship that the food wouldn't spoil or be eaten by bugs until the next growing season."

He continued as gigantic, sweaty Azerbaijani men occasionally lumbered behind him across the screen. "Nobody ever has these conversations because they're so disconnected from food and the food supply chain," he said. "People think that meat and fresh cucumbers just fucking magically appear. And, let's face it, pop nutritionists can get a lot more clicks and sell a lot more books by convincing people that food is toxic.

"But," he continued. "I *think* you're really wondering about *junk* food. Does that sound right? People conflate 'processed' with 'junk.'"

"Yes!" I said, relieved to be out of the hot seat.

"Processed food is not always junk, but junk is usually processed. I do think junk food is unhealthy, but it's not because sugar is 'toxic' or any of that nonsense," he said. "It's mainly because it's more calorie dense, less filling, and is more likely to lead someone to overeat and gain weight. And being overweight or obese is one of the largest risk factors for disease."

The rest of the conversation went that way: He led me to discover where my assumptions lay and how I relied on popular, scare-tactic narratives about food for legitimate information. He'd then cut in half what I thought I knew and give me a practical but nuanced answer painted in gray rather than the black or white I usually heard.

I left the call feeling at once smarter and dumber. Dumber because the flaws in my old thinking had been exposed. Smarter because I'd learned to think about food in a more nuanced and helpful light.

We began talking regularly. I eventually learned that Kashey is something of a diet prodigy. He earned his BS at 17. At 23, a PhD in cellular energy transduction (basically how energy moves through living things, a foundation for understanding human nutrition and athletic performance). His IQ sits around 160. Genius level.

One expert—Krista Scott Dixon, PhD, a director at Precision Nutrition, which is the world's largest online nutrition coaching company and works with professional sports teams such as the San Antonio Spurs, Houston Rockets, and Seattle Seahawks—referred to him as a "wacky, amazing, beautiful-mind genius." Despite her years of training and working in nutrition, she personally hired Kashey. "I lost ten pounds in six months on a five-foot-tall, already reasonably fit body with good habits," said Scott Dixon. "And I've maintained that ever since."

Kashey did a stint conducting research at Phoenix's Translational Genomics Research Institute. But he's never been much of a lab guy. He's more concerned with helping real people reach radical goals. Has been since he was 13.

As a teen he'd sequester himself in a library corner reading academic journals and scientific textbooks. He'd then take that wisdom and apply it to human nutrition and performance. This helped him and his father to win bodybuilding and strongman competitions.

Whispers about this teenage brick-shithouse savant circulated. Soon Kashey was a sounding board and resource for Phoenix's underground training community.

Word spread beyond the Sonoran Desert. He became popular in national elite fitness circles—bodybuilders, strongmen, ultrarunners, triathletes, Navy SEALs, etc. "I was taking relatively fit people and turning them into absolute freaks," he said. These people went from midlevel contenders to mutants: the winners of their respective competitions. By the time he was near the end of his PhD, he was fielding calls from Olympic teams (he helped a team win 16 medals in the 2016 Olympic Games) and high-profile athletes and CEOs.

After years of regularly chatting with the man, I needed to finally travel to his home base in Austin, Texas, to meet him in person and find out what else I could glean from him. I found myself standing on his doorstep with luggage and too many questions. And there he was: six feet and 260 pounds of muscle with a shaved head and burly Viking beard. He stuck out a massive hand. Thick veins ran up his arm. He'd always looked somewhat intimidating on our video calls. But in person he was like an enforcer for the Hell's Angels.

"THE SCIENTIST IN ME WOULD ALWAYS SAY 'OK, TO FIGURE OUT HOW TO GET YOU TO point B, we must find point A,'" said Kashey, after we'd settled into his office and I asked him how he began to develop his methods, the same methods he still uses. "I've never believed that people should be doing more or new things. Continuously trying to add more stuff on top of what you're doing and constantly experimenting with shiny new things is almost never the answer. It just adds another layer of stress and complication. I believe people should be doing less and eliminating limiters to progress. It's more effective to modify the behaviors and thought patterns that are keeping you from progressing," said Kashey. "Because your progress is only as good as your most obvious limiter, right?"

With that in mind, Kashey approached a person's nutrition just like he would any other scientific experiment. By gathering data. Each person tracked and reported:

- How much and what they ate. This involved weighing all the food the person ate to know true serving sizes and, therefore, calories.

- Their typical daily routine.

- Their sleep schedule.
- Their stress and energy levels.
- Their daily weight.
- Their workouts and step counts.

"I quickly 'solved' hundreds of problems just by virtue of improving a person's awareness of their own behavior," he said. "I got the idea to do this from the Hawthorne effect," a behavioral phenomenon discovered in 1958 that describes how people change the way they act when they know they are being watched. "It's a nuisance to academic scientists looking for complete control but an integral part of my empirical science where I'm looking to give control back to people," said Kashey.

His approach quickly highlighted one of the biggest fat-loss hurdles: the gap between how much a person thinks they are eating and how much they are actually eating.

We think we understand how and why we do the things we do. Especially our daily decisions like eating. What did you eat yesterday? How much, exactly? Are you *sure*? Research consistently shows people are awful at estimating portion sizes—particularly people who have struggled with their weight. Researchers associated with the Mayo Clinic recently testified that our recall of what we ate "bear[s] little relation" to what we actually ate. But overweight people's miscalculations are, on average, 300 percent greater than thin people's. One analysis discovered that people who are at a healthy weight underestimate their daily calorie intake by 281 calories, while obese people underestimate by 717, the equivalent of a Taco Bell combo meal.

A now-famous 1992 study of overweight people who claimed to be unable to lose weight despite being utterly convinced that they were eating "just 1,000 calories a day" discovered via precise measurements that those people actually consumed double that. Which is like saying "Whoops, I ate half a pizza and forgot."

I had to ask Kashey, "Don't people think it's abnormal to weigh and track every ounce of food?"

He replied with a shrug. "I was born a scientist. I started gathering data through measuring because I was used to running experiments—that's what you do when you're trying to learn something. It never occurred to me that people would think it's odd," he said. "But consider this . . . everyone measures their food somehow. How else would you determine a portion? But they just do it subconsciously, without precision. OK, many people find it odd to measure things. Many people are also sick, fat, poor, slow, and ignorant as a result of nonmeasurement."

In 2017, I became aware of my own ignorance when for a story I turned my eating over to Kashey. I was 185 pounds and had been for a decade, despite trying nearly every approach to reduce my weight. My fitness was solid—I'd finished in the top 2 percent of some large half marathons and was decently strong. But I also wasn't as lean as I wanted to be. (Who is?) Plus, my BMI was on the higher end of healthy and my hips often hurt after long runs.

At the time I was eating the same lunch every day: a protein shake and a sliced apple with a serving of peanut butter. It was cheap, tasted good, and took zero time or effort to prepare. And I always figured it was a smart choice, delivering around 500 calories and a nice balance of carbs, fat, and protein. Then I weighed my peanut butter for the first time.

What I thought was a serving of peanut butter was actually three servings, or 600 calories. The "light lunch" I'd been eating for years delivered the caloric equivalent of a Big Mac and medium fries. "When you learn how much a serving of peanut butter actually is," said Kashey, "it is completely soul crushing."

Our ignorance paired with our access to infinite quantities of cheap, ultraprocessed food adds up. A team of NIH scientists discovered that racking up 100 extra calories a day—by burning less and/or eating more—over three years adds ten pounds to the average person. That same NIH team recently found that obesity began to skyrocket in 1978, when Americans added an average of 218 extra calories per day (mostly because we snacked more and moved less). That figure alone—the equivalent of 13 tortilla chips—they believe, is enough to explain the boom in obesity.

UNDERSTANDING A TRUE PORTION—NOT THE DIABETIC-COMA-INDUCING ONES WE IN the modern world have become accustomed to—was a critical and enlightening first step for Kashey's clients. Then it was time to peel back more layers and dive into the other data they'd tracked: those lifestyle factors such as sleep, stress, and activity levels.

Kashey knew that even though weight gain or loss is mainly driven by how much food a person eats, how much food a person eats is driven by everything that is happening in his or her life. Consider: People eat 550 more calories—a whole extra meal—after nights where they sleep just five hours versus eight, according to research conducted at the Mayo Clinic.

Another experiment found that 40 percent of people eat significantly more food when they're stressed. And they're not bingeing on wheatgrass shots. Stressed people were more likely to snack on M&Ms rather than grapes. That's thanks to another life-saving evolutionary mechanism.

Kashey explained that humans essentially have two reasons for eating. For simplicity's sake, we'll call them real hunger and reward hunger. The first is set off when the body requires food to function. It fills a physiological need. It's like the body has an empty gas tank.

The second is spurred by a psychological or environmental cue. Reward hunger turns on when the body actually needs food and is experiencing real hunger, or else we wouldn't eat. (This is like sex. If sex weren't pleasurable, we wouldn't be as driven to procreate.) But reward hunger also and more frequently pops up by itself, in the absence of real hunger. Because a clock says so, because food eases stress, because we're celebrating, or because food is simply there and why not eat it? It fills a psychological want.

Real hunger is an honest dialogue between the brain and the stomach. Our stomachs are lined with mechanoreceptors, which communicate with our brain to signal fullness. When the mechanoreceptors register that the stomach is running low on food, the stomach produces a hunger-inciting hormone called ghrelin. Meanwhile, another hormone called leptin, which plays the opposite role of ghrelin and signals that we're full, drops. Our body and mind then hammer us with discomfort—our stomach feels empty and we often become irritable, foggy, and hangry. Our body also releases the stress hormones cortisol and adrenaline, which trigger a fight-or-flight response and focus our brain on finding food.

Once we eat, our brain releases dopamine, rewarding us for the behavior. This creates a circuit in the brain that associates food with dopamine.

But many times that complex dialogue isn't so honest. Grehlin, the hunger chemical, also has a habit of spurting out when our stomach is full. Particularly when delicious, calorie-dense foods are around. This is reward hunger without real hunger: a drive to eat when we don't actually *need* food. This hunger is why we can have a big dinner, feel full, but then see dessert and suddenly have room for more.

Reward hunger played an integral part in human evolution by compelling us to eat past fullness. Our bodies could then take those extra calories and add them to our frame as fat. This means that if we ever had to go without food, something that happened often before we found ourselves surrounded by stocked pantries and restaurants, our body would burn that fat to keep itself alive. In that sense, *we* were the pantry and only by eating more than we needed for the day could we fill that pantry.* You see this behavior among most mam-

---

* This is why popular "intuitive eating" programs usually fail. Our hardwired intuition tells us to eat in a way that fattens us. "Humans are programmed to prepare for the future. More of any resource is favorable to less of any resource," said Kashey. "Overcoming that, therefore, means thinking and acting purposefully, in direct opposition to intuition." This explains why Kashey has clients track food with data rather than feelings.

mals: "Given the opportunity, a grizzly will eat until it can't move," Donnie told me. Much like modern humans at a buffet.

Our brains evolved to release more dopamine when eating calorie-packed foods (think of the pleasure of eating pecan pie versus, like, a raw piece of broccoli). This is why humans crave foods that are sweet, fatty, and/or salty. Those qualities signal that a food is an efficient way to fill our onboard pantry.

Through the broad sweep of time, reward hunger in the absence of real hunger was exceedingly healthy for humans. It kept us alive. That's because early humans had no means of storing food. Sorry, no refrigerators or freezers or Yeti coolers. Early humans also rarely knew where their next meal was coming from. And the food we ate most often wasn't exactly "comfort food," calorie-packed food that causes a surge of dopamine and tastes better than anything we could ever find in nature.*

But we're now swimming in calorie-dense, craveable eats our ancestors didn't have. Like formulated, ready-to-eat, multiple ingredient foods that go through hundreds of iterations, based on laboratory testing and consumer feedback, to be delicious and bingeable. These are foods that mix carbs and fat, like ice cream, baked goods, cheeseburgers, chips, pizza, etc. Fast food and packaged food sales rose roughly 25 and 10 percent in America over the last five years.

The carb-fat combo doesn't exist naturally, but it's one that humans clamor for, say scientists at Yale. Researchers at the NIH explain our new trouble with reward hunger this way: "In evolutionary terms, this property of palatable foods used to be advantageous in environments where food sources were scarce and/or unreliable because it ensured that food was eaten when available, enabling energy to be stored in the body (as fat) for future use. However, in societies

---

* Conversely, maybe all food was comfort food, in the sense that it is comfortable to not starve and die.

like ours, where food is plentiful and ubiquitous, this adaptation has become a dangerous liability."*

THE SURGE OF COMFORTING DOPAMINE CAUSED BY FOOD ALSO EXPLAINS WHY WE

can eat to alleviate discomforts ranging from stress to sadness to boredom. "Comfort food" and "stress eating" are common American vernacular, and studies show that real hunger now drives just 20 percent of eating. The rate at which the people in the study ate was so astounding that it led the research team to wonder if people ever eat when they're actually hungry anymore.

Consider the Covid-19 quarantines. Many experienced significant weight gain while shuttered inside for months. Not just from being less active, but also from seeking calm and comfort—and food was a cheap and easy way to deal with the stress.

The "Quarantine 15" and much of our modern weight gain are driven by a phenomenon discovered by scientists at the University of Pennsylvania. The researchers found that when people do eat for reasons other than real hunger, they're far more likely to binge past fulfillment into a dazed-and-doughy state of psychic sedation.

The cliché of the person who mows through an entire pint of ice cream after a breakup? It's real. But the phenomenon also plays out every day in much smaller ways. A few pieces of candy from the office jar when we have a deadline. Seconds of dinner (even something we think is healthy or that fits our fad diet) after a long day at work. Gluttonous food and drinks to celebrate a win.

"This is why I would much rather address the question 'Why are you eating?' versus 'Eat this food at this time,'" said Kashey.

"We've all been taught to eat when we are hungry," said Ashley Bunge, a successful 49-year-old client of Kashey's. She came to him

---

* Before the Industrial Revolution, being significantly overweight was even more of a liability because you couldn't work, produce, or contribute.

morbidly obese, diabetic, unable to walk more than half a block, and having tried every diet ever. Her next option was bypass surgery. "I would always snack because I thought I was *starving* all the time. Kashey taught me that hunger can be deceptive. I learned I often just had a psychological need to eat. He taught me that it's okay to be hungry. My response was 'WHAT???' He told me to 'embrace the suck.' Now, yeah, I'm hungry sometimes. It is what it is. I'm OK with being uncomfortable now. I remind myself that I'm safe, have food, and will eat when it's time to eat."

She's down about 150 pounds and still losing. "I swim, lift weights, hike, walk miles at a time, and am off my medications," said Bunge.

Kashey told me Bunge's story is one he's seen thousands of times. In middle-aged saleswomen, professional athletes, Special Forces soldiers, CEOs . . . you name it.

"People who are at a consistently healthy weight don't have better genetics or a higher metabolism, and they don't magically burn more calories," he said. "They're just more likely to deal with stress by, like, going for a walk instead of eating. That's really the difference." More research has backed up this claim, finding that uncontrollable factors like metabolic dysfunction are exceedingly rare. The science suggests that genes may play a role in obesity. But these genes seem to move the dial only when they meet our new laziness-inducing, food-filled environment. We didn't used to get fat, and our genes haven't changed.*

"If you have these low-level stressors all the time that you deal with by taking candy from the candy jar, that adds up. Or maybe you have one super-stressful event per month that you handle by eating a massive burger, fries, and milkshake," he said. "Ten years later you'll

---

* Kashey explained his thoughts on obesity genes like this: "Whether or not you have some obesity gene, you treat the condition in the exact same way you would if you didn't have that gene. You eat better and move more. So why are we even talking about this?" he said. "Is it perhaps harder for some people to lose weight than others? Maybe. Will those people have to work harder? Maybe. But life isn't fair, and by harping on genes, people just give themselves an excuse to fail."

probably find yourself ten or twenty pounds heavier. Many people today don't know how to deal with stress. They are neither hardy nor resilient, and they have no shortage of comfort food to distract themselves from stress."

When I worked with Kashey, for example, I noticed that I would come home from work on Friday and be drawn to the pantry by my wife's bulk-size bag of kettle corn or peanut M&Ms. When I brought this up with Kashey, he had no advice, just a question: "What happens on Friday?"

"Well, I get home from work earlier . . . and I usually sit in the kitchen and send some final emails, and then I feel like the week is done, and . . ." Bingo. I was using food to reward myself and offload the week's stress.

He recommended that I distract the discomfort of reward hunger with another form of discomfort: light exercise. "Find some 'calorie negative' ways of dealing with stress," he said. "Walking is my number one. It relieves more stress and is health promoting. It leads you to burn calories rather than onboard them. And it removes you from the situation and adds time for reflection, where you can realize that you weren't really hungry."

MORE RESEARCH IS LENDING SCIENTIFIC CREDIT TO WHAT KASHEY HAS PROVED TIME and time again in the real world. Dr. Marc Potenza holds an MD and a PhD and is a professor of psychiatry at Yale. He's now on the editorial board of 15 academic journals, has penned more than 600 studies, and has been cited nearly 40,000 times. He's the type of fastidious scientist you want researching what could be the next big breakthrough in obesity.

"I'm interested in understanding the behaviors that can be potentially harmful for people," he told me. "And I've long been interested in eating behavior. So if one thinks about the public health impacts of certain behaviors, which are the most impactful? Obesity and smoking vie for what's associated with the most morbidity and mortality in the general population."

Potenza is considered one of the world's foremost experts on why people engage in harmful behaviors, like pathological gambling. And in that research—hundreds of studies—he discovered that stress is a key trigger that leads people to pull the slot handle, make the sports bet, or buy the scratch-off lottery ticket. He wondered if stress might work the same way with food, causing us to shuttle junk into our mouths.

To find out, he read hundreds of studies on the topic of stress and if it changes how and what we eat, and how that might explain our current, collective ability to tip scales unlike any other time in our 2.5-million-year history. The answer: Undoubtedly, yes.

We face two kinds of stress: acute and chronic. Acute stress is an alarm response, like a "jump scare" in a horror movie. Our heart pounds, blood pressure rises, and adrenaline spurts out. Blood is shuttled to our limbs, heart, and brain so we can either fight or flee. Chronic stress is less intense but long-lasting. It results in the sustained, slow drip of a different hormone, called cortisol.

Humans and other primates are uniquely predisposed to chronic stress. That's because we're smart, social creatures who have a lot of downtime to be "miserable to each other and stress each other out," according to Robert Sapolsky, the Stanford neuroendocrinologist and recipient of a MacArthur "Genius" grant.

Our modern world doesn't have conventional, acute stressors like, as Sapolsky put it, "getting done in by predators." We instead create and propagate chronic stressors—keeping up with the Joneses, work drama, bills, gossip, that kind of thing. Which is why we are now, Sapolsky said, getting done in by ourselves. By the tales we tell ourselves about what we need to achieve and when and why and in relation to whom.

The slow drip of cortisol from chronic stress not only kickstarts reward eating in many people but also erodes their self-restraint. This creates "a potent formula for obesity," wrote Potenza. "[Because] food is an inexpensive resource for providing . . . short-term pleasure and relief from discomfort."

One study found that overweight people are more likely to eat when faced with stress compared to lean people. Another found that, even when they weren't hungry, overweight people reported having more food cravings and eating more junk foods. Potenza in his research wrote that "given the rewarding properties of food, it is hypothesized that hyperpalatable foods may serve as 'comfort food' that acts as a form of self-medication" to distract people from unwanted stress.

Ultraprocessed foods are like cheap, over-the-counter, omnipresent Xanax. But, as with pills, once the effect wears off, the stress is still there. So a person must then take another pill or eat more junk. Side effects? Weight gain, heart disease, stroke, cancer, high blood pressure, high LDL cholesterol, type-2 diabetes, fatigue, depression, osteoarthritis, pain, early death, etc.

Stress eating also, according to Potenza, is why most restrictive fad diets fail. Potenza points to a highly influential study conducted by scientists in the UK. It found that fad dieters who faced heavy work stress crumpled and ate the foods that were off-limits, while their coworkers who weren't fad dieters didn't eat any differently when stressed. The all-or-nothing approach seems to make the off-limits foods more attractive and rewarding. Other research shows that people are less likely to comply with health-promoting programs the more stress they face.

Fad diets also, according to a seminal 1989 study, mess with a person's ability to gauge their hunger. The researchers discovered that people who have rigid food rules are less in tune with their body's cues of hunger and fullness, which leads them to overeat far past fullness. Conversely, dieters who were more flexible and didn't ban foods were less likely to go off the rails and binge, according to other research.*

---

* More factors could be at play. Perhaps the same type of person who jumps on a fad diet also has less impulse control. And maybe people who aren't in tune with hunger feel a

The triggers that lead a person to stress eat—the stressors—are inevitable. But a person *can* upgrade the resulting behavior. Harvard scientists pointed to changing personal behaviors as the number-one way to prevent obesity. That means strengthening ourselves to deal with discomfort in a different way.

BEYOND THE HOW MUCH AND WHY A PERSON IS EATING, KASHEY ALSO USES HUNGER to guide the what—the actual foods a person eats—in an unconventional way. First off, he teaches that no foods are off-limits.

"Kashey helped me remove the morality, guilt, and emotion from my nutrition decision making," said a Navy SEAL who is a client of Kashey's. The client needed to be incredibly strong but also light enough that he could move in on targets quickly. The problem was that he had established good and evil food rules, and he'd often give in to intense reward hunger stemming from stress and emotion. In those instances he'd binge on junk, setting himself back significantly. This is a common phenomenon called the disinhibition effect, and researchers at the NIH found that it caused a group of overly restrictive dieters to go through a roller coaster of gains and losses over six years, ending with their being heavier than when they started.

But on Kashey's plan the SEAL could eat anything, including junk foods, as long as he stayed within his daily calorie goals.* "I learned to remove emotion and morality from decision making and instead let the data guide me," he said. "I've racked up a lot of improvements. Kashey started me on this path with nutrition, but soon

---

greater need to try to exert control over it with rigid rules. Either way, the problem lies in how we cope.

* For their first week working with Kashey, a client would track everything they normally did and ate. Once he had the person's data, Kashey would compare it to established academic literature and calculate the person's food requirements based on his or her size, activity level, and current weight, giving the person a specific number of calories and protein to eat. Clients were still required to track everything they did and ate, and send him weekly data. "How else would they know if they were sticking to the plan?" he says. He'd then make subtle weekly tweaks, which he called "dynamic adjustment," unlike other diets, where the plan is the plan and it doesn't change.

I was applying these lessons to every area of my life and watching wins pile up."

Kashey indeed has no food ideology. "I don't care what people eat," he said. "Just so long as they keep track of it." Consistently leveraging the Hawthorne effect.

Of course, he said, junk foods come with a tradeoff. Not all foods are created equal when it comes to mitigating reward hunger and fending off disinhibition eating. "A lot of new clients take advantage of the fact that all foods are acceptable, it's just about moderating the amounts. So they'll eat, like, pizza for breakfast, lunch, and dinner. But then they realize that two thousand or two thousand five hundred calories in pizza is not filling them up. Because pizza is so calorie dense. They can't eat enough to stay full while staying within their calorie constraints. They become miserably hungry eating that way."

"Then why don't you just tell people to not eat junk?" I asked.

"Because if I say 'Hey, you shouldn't eat pizza,' then the person is just going to resent me and turn into a ticking pizza time bomb," he said, echoing Potenza's research showing that people who have rigid all-or-nothing rules around food are more likely to, like the SEAL, ditch a healthy diet and eat far beyond fullness, typically setting them back even further than when the diet started. "But if I say 'Eat what you feel like eating, bro. Go for it, have a blast—just stay within your plan,' then it becomes a learning opportunity. Then people come back to me and are like, 'Dr. Kashey, I followed the plan eating entirely pizza and I'm starving.' So then my reply is 'Great. Tell me what other foods you enjoy that you think will keep you satisfied longer.'"

Hunger is necessary for long-term weight loss. But there's a growing recognition that mitigating it could improve our success. And going for a walk to stave off hunger can only work to a point. Scientists in Australia wondered how foods differed in their ability to make a person feel full. Their hypothesis was that eating foods that are more filling per calorie would satisfy a person before they accidentally overate.

To test the theory, the researchers chose 38 common foods. There were four different fruits, five different baked goods, seven different snacks, six different high-protein foods, nine different carb-heavy foods, and seven different breakfast cereals.

Participants arrived in the morning, before breakfast. They then ate a 240-calorie serving of one of the 38 foods and reported their hunger levels every 15 minutes for 2 hours. Afterward they went to a breakfast buffet, where the researchers tracked every morsel of food the participants subsequently ate. The experiment was repeated often, with the same participants trying a variety of the foods. (The scientists didn't include vegetables because vegetables aren't a staple food, meaning 240 calories of, for example, broccoli would equate to 12 servings of broccoli, an amount that no one actually eats in a meal.)

Foods differed by as much as 700 percent in their ability to fight hunger. Each subject ate the same amount of calories initially. But the subjects eating the more filling foods then ate less at the buffet later on—their calories went further or shorter depending on their food earlier on.

The least filling food was croissants, while the most filling was plain white potatoes. The USDA reports that a small croissant and a medium potato both have about 170 calories. This study suggests you'd have to eat about seven croissants, 1,190 calories, to experience the same fullness you'd get from a single potato. The key quality that made a food filling: how heavy its 240-calorie serving size was.

Kashey thinks of this as the "energy density" of a food and uses it to help his clients transcend hunger. It leverages our ancestral eating patterns to help us understand real hunger, mitigate reward hunger, improve health, and boost performance. It's the same method he used to feed the medal-winning Olympians he coached.

It's easiest to think about this concept as the amount of energy or calories per pound of a given food. "So, for example, at one end of the spectrum there's something like iceberg lettuce. There are sixty calories in a pound of iceberg lettuce. At the extreme opposite end of the spectrum there are oils, like olive oil or canola oil. A pound of oil has four thousand calories," Kashey explained. "When you're making a direct comparison of these foods, there's about a six thousand five hundred percent difference in how many calories a pound of these foods have." Every other food we eat lies between these two foods. Junk food such as chips, candy bars, desserts, and even energy bars, for example, have about 2,000 calories per pound. Processed grains like breads and crackers have about 1,500, while unprocessed grains like cooked rice and oats have 500. Tubers, fruits, and vegetables have about 400, 300, and 120, respectively.

"The reason I belabor this concept with my clients is because of those mechanoreceptors in our stomachs that communicate with our brains to signal fullness," Kashey said. "Pretend that in a perfect world it takes one pound of food for these mechanoreceptors to be happy. You can see how a person could leverage this to be full on fewer calories."

"Let's say a person wants to eat two thousand calories over four meals. That's five hundred calories a meal," said Kashey. For example, if a person were to eat only olive oil for one meal, it would be just a shot glass of oil. "That's enough energy to fuel your body," he said. "But because that oil takes up so little room in your stomach you're going to be left hungry. Of course, no one eats olive oil for lunch, but you get the point.

"So a lot of people will think, 'OK, I'll just eat the lowest-density items. Tons of vegetables and fresh fruit and I'll be full and lose weight,'" said Kashey. "But the body isn't stupid. Remember, the brain communicates with the stomach. So the body knows something is in our stomach, but does that something have enough energy to power you? Your brain eventually figures out that your stomach is full of stuff that's not giving it enough energy to function properly." This is another defense mechanism that kept our species alive. Without it, every time we got hungry we could have eaten, say, mud and been satisfied—while eventually starving to death.

"So you lose weight—until your brain responds by sending out mega-cravings for calorie-dense items," said Kashey. "And that leads to bingeing, which leads to weight gain, paradoxically." Again, the disinhibition effect.

"The question then becomes, What *should* a person eat? What combinations of foods are optimal? Because you can't eat just one food, and people rarely have just one food group on a plate," said Kashey.

The World Cancer Research Fund/American Institute of Cancer Research (WCRF/AICR) has spent three decades analyzing all the data on cancer prevention. They release a massive report each decade, and their most recent one stated that "cancer is a multifactorial disease that is fueled by a deranged metabolism." Which is why they concluded that being at a healthy weight was the number-one thing a person could do to prevent cancer.

Naturally, the WCRF/AICR then wondered what types of foods people could eat to maintain a healthy, disease-resistant body weight. So they analyzed the dietary data of tens of thousands of people. "I read the report," said Kashey. "The number they tabulated was food that has about five hundred sixty-seven calories per pound. The exactitude of the number is meaningless. But the practical takeaway is important: A person should mostly be eating unprocessed whole grains* and tubers, fruits and vegetables, and lowish-fat animal protein." These foods lead us to the sweet spot where we find a healthy weight and keep meal satisfaction high, he said. "An average plate could be a quarter animal protein, a quarter whole grains or tubers, and half vegetables or fruit. Highly active people might want to do

---

* Unprocessed whole grains are grains that must be cooked in water before we can eat them. Think: rice, oatmeal, quinoa, etc. Their energy density (calories per pound) is taken after cooking.

half whole grains or tubers and a quarter vegetables or fruit." (A number of Kashey's clients said they'll also add calorie-light foods like cabbage or spinach to their meals, to make them even more filling.)

It's a combo of food that doctors, governments, and major health organizations have advocated for years. It's also one that's at odds with most fad diets: It's not low carb or low fat. It's not vegan or paleo. "It's eating like a fucking adult," said Kashey. And, importantly, not eating ourselves into supreme comfort each meal.

Kashey's logic behind why it works is what makes his approach innovative. Because the foods are so healthful and filling, the body better checks reward hunger and naturally finds the right amount to eat. And a person can fit delicious, dopamine-spiking junk food into his method without guilt or fear of weight gain. They just have to accept that they'll likely be hungrier later. This approach respects the idea that foods, after all, are not just vehicles for delivering energy. Foods are often a connection to family, community, culture, and identity, and should never be off-limits.

The method has been validated in the lab. A team of leading researchers at the NIH, for example, found that people placed on a high-energy-density diet naturally ate 500 more calories each day and gained weight while those on the lower-density diet like Kashey's lost weight.

The phenomenon has also played out in the real world for thousands of years. Just consider the Kitavans.

In the early 1990s, the Swedish anthropologist Staffan Lindeberg traveled to the island of Kitava, in Papua New Guinea. He was there studying the Kitavan people, a traditional society largely uninfluenced by Western lifestyle. These are people living somewhere between hunter-gatherers and subsistence farmers. Lindeberg wrote, "Cultivated tubers (mainly yam, sweet potato and taro) are staples, supplemented by fruits, leaves, [coconuts], fish, maize, tapioca and beans." All less calorically dense foods, save for the occasional coconut. About 70 percent of their calories come from carbohydrates—so you could say the Kitavans have a high-carb diet—and they eat around 2,200 calories a day, despite having plenty of food in storage.

Critically, Lindeberg reported, the Kitavans eat no processed, higher-density foods. He found no overweight Kitavans and zero indications of heart disease or evidence that any Kitavan had ever had a heart attack or stroke. The majority of people he tested were over 50 years old. A handful even reached past 90—quite a feat without modern medicine. Meanwhile, in his home country of Sweden, nearly half of the people were overweight or obese, and heart disease and strokes were the top killers. Diet was seemingly the answer.

Lindeberg's was a finding that's been repeated often: People who eat a diet that focuses on whole foods experience less disease. The Tsimane people, a tribe in Bolivia, eat rice, plantains, tubers, and corn; meat and fish that they themselves hunt and pull from streams; fruit; and the occasional wild nuts. They register the healthiest hearts ever recorded, according to a global team of scientists. The chronic-disease-free Hadza, in Tanzania, eat mostly wild tubers, fruits, and meats. These general rules also apply to modern industrial societies that eat fewer higher-density foods. The people of Japan are some of the longest living and least likely to die from heart disease and cancer in the developed world, a fact researchers partially credit to their traditional diet of rice, lean proteins, and vegetables.

That a diet based primarily on tubers and whole grains is "good for you" goes against the advice of every low-carb diet—from paleo to keto to Atkins—pop nutrition stories, and even academic institutions like Harvard. Bunge told me that she "actually cried a couple times when [Kashey] suggested I eat more carbs, because my past with dieting had made me think that's what was making me fat."

Consider the plain white potato. Harvard's nutrition department recommends people stay away from potatoes, citing studies that show people who increased their consumption of French fries gained 3.4 pounds over four years.

I told Kashey that and he laughed. "Only somebody with multiple advanced degrees could say something that stupid," he said. "That's like banning screwdrivers because guns have screws in them."

Indeed, the problem—as with all foods that come from the earth—is with us and our drive to turn natural foods into dopamine-jacking comfort foods. Take how we ruin the nutrition packed into potatoes. We cut them into little sticks or paper-thin wafers, then bathe them in heated cooking oil (50 percent of America's potatoes go to fries, chips, and other "potato products"). Or we boil them, then mash them with butter and cream. We bake them, then slather them with more butter, sour cream, and—depending on how far south a person finds herself—cheese and fatty, saucy meats. These treatments spike a food's energy density. "In other words," said Kashey, "it's no longer a potato. It's a vessel for gluttony." A pound of French fries, for example, has an energy density of more than 1,500, compared to just 400 for a pound of plain baked potatoes.

In my four months working with Kashey, the Hawthorne effect took full effect. I became aware of how, why, and what I was eating. I dropped 15 pounds, to 170 pounds. My running times plummeted. I was just as strong (which meant I was actually stronger pound-for-pound). I had more energy and my hip pain went away. When I sent Kashey progress pictures he said I looked "like some secret agent human weapon."

I was hungry, of course, but I implemented Kashey's methods. And eventually the hunger faded. Not only do the body's hunger chemicals normalize after the internal shock of the initial weight loss, but we also expand our comfort zone and realize hunger isn't an emergency. "Real hunger is seldom the real issue compared to the desire to eat," said Kashey.

Before I left Austin, I thought of my conversation with Potenza. I asked Kashey if he thought people were more stressed now than in the past.

"Yeah, I don't know. Probably? It seems so," he said. "Although I think it depends on what kind of stress we're talking about, because there is one stress we face far less of."

"What's that?" I asked.

"Stress from lean times," he said. "We no longer have times where we go without food, which cause us to have a period where we'd naturally lose weight."

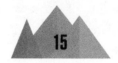

15

12 TO 16 HOURS

HUMANS EVOLVED IN a landscape of feast and famine. Our weight vacillated with the seasons and what nature offered to us. Thankfully we've mostly lost the forced famine. But we now seemingly have only two variations of feasting. We're either kind of feasting, where we maintain our weight, or we're definitely feasting, where we add weight. Hunger is missing from our daily, weekly, monthly, and yearly wellness prescription.

Rarely feeling real hunger is a strong sign that a person is suffering from the ill effects of comfort creep, according to a surge of new scientific evidence.

The data shows that we don't typically gain weight in a linear fashion, like a quarter pound each month for a total of three pounds at the end of the year. Most of us maintain our weight most of the year, then experience periods of gain, according to a study in the *New England Journal of Medicine*. Scientists have identified big stressors, like getting married, moving, and the holidays, as times where people are most likely to pack on pounds.* For example, the subjects in the study didn't gain much weight in the fall before Thanksgiving or in

---

* We often frame stress as always negative. But stress can also be positive, such as celebrations.

the months after the New Year. They did, however, put on anywhere from one to five holiday pounds. And the critical point was that the participants never lost that weight.

Anthropologists and historians know that our ancestors experienced persistent hunger. But despite what some paleo diet books will have us believe, early humans likely didn't go for extended stretches without a single calorie. A day at most. And that was rare, according to food historians at Yale.

But it *is* agreed that these people weren't eating around the clock. The research suggests they likely ate one or two meals a day. And between meals they surely weren't snacking on vending-machine foods or sipping Frappuccinos.

Most modern people, on the other hand, start cramming in calories upon waking up and don't stop until right before bed, Satchin Panda, PhD, a scientist at the Salk Institute for Biological Studies, explained. One of Panda's studies found that the average person now eats across a 15-hour window. Research from the University of North Carolina discovered that we're snacking 75 percent more than we were before 1978. Our snacks are also 60 percent larger and more likely to be ultraprocessed.

The effects of this consistent stream of sugar, salt, and fat and our two versions of feasting are compounded over time, wrote the researchers in the *New England Journal of Medicine* study. "As this gain is not reversed during spring or summer months," they concluded, "[this] weight gain appears likely to contribute to the increase in body weight that frequently occurs during adulthood." Our growing disconnection from hunger is one of the critical reasons obesity began its rocket-like rise in the late 1970s.

Beyond weight, the trouble with rarely feeling real hunger is that our bodies evolved to leverage lean times for good. Lean times are, in fact, a necessary state for optimizing long-term health. This is because a hungry human body undergoes a sort of cellular natural selection.

We fully metabolize our last meal after 12 to 16 hours, depending on how much we ate. That's when our body releases testosterone, adrenaline, and cortisol: a symphony of hormones that act as signals to burn stored tissues for energy. But we don't burn our finest tissues. "We get rid of a lot of dead and damaged cells," said Panda.

Humans have tinkered with hunger as a way to enter a new dimension of religious experience, biological revision, and physical metamorphosis for thousands of years, said Adrienne Rose Bitar, PhD, a historian at Cornell. Medical minds ranging from Hippocrates in 500 BC to American doctors in the 1800s, for example, theorized that stretches without food could help prevent and even fight back against diseases like cancer. In the early 1990s we figured out why there may be a nugget of truth in these old claims.

In 1992, David Sabatini, PhD, MD, a biologist at MIT, discovered what's called the mTOR pathway. He told me to think of it as a general contractor, signaling to the body to demolish its old cells and replace them with newer, healthier ones. The body's oldest cells have all sorts of problems and are implicated in many of the diseases that end up killing us.

"You couldn't fully renovate the old house by bringing in only a plumber, or only an electrician or roofer or drywall guy," he said. "You'd need to hire a general contractor, who would hire all those specialists, who would then come fix all those problems that needed to be fixed."

The mTOR pathway senses whether your body is fed or not fed. When you go without food the contractor calls in all his workers. "It's the one way you can trigger a whole series of events that are rejuvenating and antiaging," said Sabatini. Your body is ruthlessly efficient, and it culls the herd by consuming your oldest, weakest cells. A researcher at Cedars-Sinai Medical Center calls this process your body's way of "taking out the trash."

These trash cells are ones that no longer divide and are thought to drive aging and disease. A study in *Nature* said that these cells "disrupt normal tissue function." They cause inflammation, kill healthy cells, induce fibrosis, and inhibit the function of beneficial growth cells. These trash cells "actively damage the tissues in which they reside and can be directly linked to features of natural aging," said the scientists. They're also associated with cancer, Alzheimer's, infections, osteoarthritis, excessive blood sugar and blood lipid levels, and more.

The body's "taking out the trash" process is officially called autophagy, which translates from ancient Greek as "self-devouring." Autophagy is, in many ways, a metaphor for what happens to all things under discomfort: Our weak links—whether physical or psychological—are painfully sacrificed for our good.

Humans probably developed autophagy in concert with day and night cycles, generating what Panda calls circadian rhythms. The research suggests that the body has programmed within it a code to crank up autophagy to repair and rejuvenate itself at night, as it burns through the day's food.

But our 15-hour daily eating windows disrupt the process, said Panda. They rob our bodies of the 12 to 16 hours we need to fully metabolize food and lapse into autophagy mode. Or, as the Cedars Sinai scientist put it, "If you eat . . . before bed, you're not going to have any autophagy. That means you're not going to take out the trash, so the cells begin to accumulate more and more debris."

A team of scientists from 16 different institutions including Harvard and Johns Hopkins who studied the topic wrote, "For many of our ancestors, food was probably scarce and primarily consumed during daylight hours, leaving long hours of overnight fasting. With the advent of affordable artificial lighting and industrialization, modern humans began to experience prolonged hours of illumination every day and resultant extended consumption of food."

Daily eating marathons also may have caused us to lose a step in our mental game. Somewhat paradoxically, a lack of food typically leads to a surge of energy. "The ability to function at a high level, both physically and mentally, during our extended periods without food may have been of fundamental importance in our evolutionary history," wrote that team of scientists. This is likely why we often define the word "hunger" as not just discomfort from a lack of food but also as ambitious drive. It's a drive that crosses animalistic distinctions.

"During [extended time without food], the body doesn't shut down, it ramps up," Dr. Jason Fung, a nephrologist and author of *The Obesity Code,* told me. "Think about a hungry wolf versus a lion who just ate. Which one is more focused? The hungry wolf."

According to researchers at the University of Southern California, these advantageous responses to hunger first appeared billions of years ago in prokaryotes, microscopic single-celled organisms that were the first life on earth.

Recall the human hunger response of spurting hormones and burning fat. This gives the body energy from fat and from adrenaline, and adrenaline has been shown to increase alertness and focus, said Fung.

Today we don't have to worry about needing the energy and mental acuity to, say, run down, track, and kill a dik-dik. But we can still leverage hunger's evolutionary chemical upsides to conquer our more modern goals. Hunger may help humans be more focused and productive in the tasks of modern life, according to Panda and Fung. Other research shows that people who stop eating a few hours before bed sleep better, said Panda. "So if you sleep longer and deeper, you're likely to be more focused the next day."

All this research is at odds with fad diet marketing, which has programmed us to ask, "What should I eat?" when we want to improve our health. Going without food and feeling some real hunger is often far more powerful.

We're told, for example, that breakfast is the most important meal of the day (often in studies funded by, say, cereal companies). Yet little scientific evidence shows that it has any benefit over any other meal, according to research in the *American Journal of Clinical Nutrition.*

And simply nixing breakfast hits the "sweet spot for practicality" in reacquainting a person with hunger, said Panda. It allows the body to go 12 to 16 hours without a calorie, which goes "a long way toward preventing diseases, increasing alertness and energy," said Panda. And if a person eats a reasonable lunch they can enjoy a good-size dinner without worrying too much about gaining weight. Getting off breakfast often sucks at first. But that's only because the body and mind take time to adapt to change and initially miss sucking down food upon wake-up.

Other research shows that programming two "hungry days" per week where we eat around 500 calories delivers benefits. A study in the *International Journal of Obesity* found that six months of this method led to more than 10 pounds of weight loss and health improvements in obese people. The catch is that a person can't go crazy and pound food on their regular eating days.

Another option is to string together five "hungry days" in a row, once a month, eating just 700 total calories. A study in *Cell Metabolism* found that approach helped rejuvenate aging organs and increase the health span of mice.

And researchers at Harvard report that occasional 24-hour stints without food can help reduce our appetite during our normal eating hours. This decreases average levels of insulin, a hormone that may determine the body's "set weight." The researchers also say these longer fasts may better stimulate cleaning out our old cells.

Rewilding our eating habits won't be easy. It requires that we step back and become aware of how much and why we're eating. It requires us to favor the foods humans have eaten for thousands of years but not be afraid of or feel guilty for the occasional comfort food.

Of utmost importance, it requires that we embrace the discomfort of hunger. We must recognize that occasionally going without food up to 24 hours is a normal and even beneficial human state. And we must also understand and adapt to the fact that much of our hunger isn't real physiological hunger. Rather, it's often a cheap coping mechanism to comfort us against the discomforts of modern life.

WILLIAM WAS A BIRD OF PREY AS WE HIKED, ALWAYS SEARCHING FOR MICROSCOPIC shards of off-white caribou chests against pockets of snow and muted earth. We're now stopped on a hill a few miles from camp and his eye is entirely in the scope. No chatting.

Donnie's sitting on the damp ground, legs unfurled, binoculars to his face.

The weather's shit. If it isn't snowing or sprinkling, then it's freezing cold. If I want to sit, I do so on the half-frozen ground. The cold has a way of making me even more ravenous, as my body cranks through calories to fuel its internal furnaces.

Arctic-induced misery has been omnipresent in one way or another since we put boots to ground. But this morning I recalled a line that's helped me stay sober—"And acceptance is the answer to all my problems today"—and applied it to my current condition. I quit fighting the elements, hunger, landscape, etc.

"How you doing?" asks Donnie.

"I'm good!" I respond, surprising myself with my positivity.

Donnie smiles and shakes his head approvingly. "I have a lot of friends who proclaim to love the wilderness and spending time in it," he says. "But what they consider wild is skiing at a resort all day, then going to the lodge for a vodka and a cheeseburger. Or hunting at a retreat with luxury cabins. There's absolutely no shame in that. But I think there's more charm in what we're doing. And I think the experiences out here affect you much differently and deeply."

He continues. "I recently read this book. . . . It's proven the harder you work for something, the happier you'll be about it," he says. He's referring to NYU researcher Jonathan Haidt's work *The Happiness Hypothesis*. And here I thought I was the nerd on the trip.

Williams spots a herd across the valley.

"How far?" asks Donnie.

"Far."

We see caribou often but almost never up close. And therein lies the problem.

More weather rolls in. This area is characterized by fits of sun and storm. Sometimes our view is clear. Other times the misty clouds are either above us, below us, to the side of us, or engulfing us. And so it is with the caribou, who use this weather to their advantage. The small herd William sees is swallowed by the mist. And when it clears 20 minutes later—abracadabra—the animals are nowhere to be seen.

Despite moments of misery, I'm enjoying myself. The actual hunting part, however, is starting to feel like a fool's errand. The animals are too smart, too paranoid, and too tuned in to every happening within a few hundred yards of them. And we, it seems, are too ignorant to realize this.

We spend more time watching, move positions, and watch more.

"Not a fuckin' one," says William, folding the scope.

In a last-ditch effort to spot caribou we climb shale cliffs to the top of a 1,000-foot-high butte. The rock slides from its sides in a deluge of half-inch-thick wafers that skim downhill as we climb. Up here we can see in every direction. A peregrine falcon hovers high overhead, waiting to make its 200-mile-an-hour dive-bomb onto unsuspecting prey.

We circumvent the top of the butte, looking for white dots in the surrounding valleys. Nothing. We sit on the loose chalk and flat shale flakes, springing from which are brown flowers, neon lichen, and caribou moss. Life persists.

When the sun begins to dip we traverse back down the cliff. William's first, I'm second, then it's Donnie, who pauses for a few minutes midway down the face.

He addresses this pause once we convene at the bottom. "You know, boys, I stood up on that treacherous hill for a moment. I thought about our failure. I thought about everything wrong with the world.

I thought about how entropy was bringing me and everything I love closer to death and decay each second. And it was all very heavy." He pauses. "But then I thought . . . well"—a shit-eating grin slides across his face—"the good news is that we have Mountain House dinners back at the teepee. So I've got that going for me."

William shakes his head. I'm doubled over.

I'm hungry as we hike back to camp. Not just for food. Also for life. My worldview has encountered a sea change. I've found a quiet awareness of the world around me and rediscovered lost sensations. One of my favorite parts of the recent days is when we walk quietly back to camp with the sun setting. It's experiencing the Arctic as it goes through its own circadian rhythms, entering into itself for the night. Birds nesting, animals heading into their burrows, a cold silence and stillness setting in.

PART FOUR

Think about your death every day.

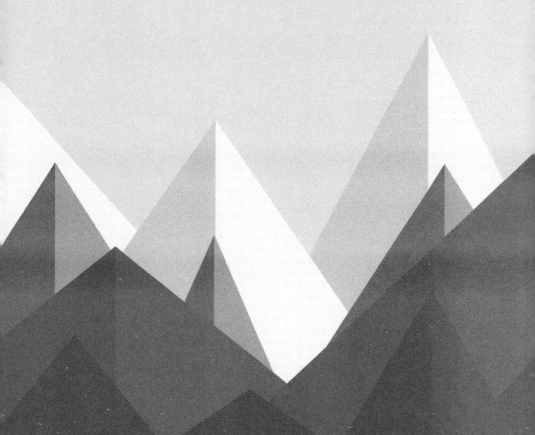

16

3 GOOD LEGS

THE EVENING AFTER our hike to the top of the butte, we sat inside the teepee and concluded that perhaps the great caribou highway had been diverted past us.

So the next morning we packed camp, inciting a newfound energy into our group. "Time for a move! Ti-i-ime for a fuuh-uuh-uuh-ckin' moo-oo-oove!" sang William as he rolled his sleeping pad and bag and shoved gear into his pack. We headed a good 20 miles north, to a river valley flanked by two ancient hills. There we made camp on a hillside opposite that valley, so that we could stay out of sight and smell of the herds moving through it.

Our new camp is a steep, quad-burning hike to the top of the ridge, which is about a tenth of a mile wide and all shale, until it slopes off into tundra tussocks and rocky grass, running downhill at a 15-degree pitch. We're now sitting below the ridgetop. This position keeps us high enough to view the entire valley and opposite hill, yet we blend into the land and are out of caribou sight lines. They're wary of little black dots on the horizon.

The valley and its surrounding hills are a wide bowl with few harsh angles or sharp surfaces, like a Grand Canyon worn soft and wide by time. After a mile our hill flattens into a two-mile-wide valley that mixes river, tundra, frosty swamp, and thickets of five-foot-tall willows. Passageways run through the thickets, escape routes created by animals across millennia. The land then climbs up into another hill.

And there is currently a "lotta caribou on that hill," says William, sitting in a patch of shale, the spotting scope propped between his splayed-out legs. "One looks like a shooter."

A light breeze pushes the valley's soft, milky scent uphill and into my nose. I'm using an oversize tussock as a stool. Donnie is using one as a backrest. "Let me see," says Donnie, lurching up from his seat.

William pulls back his head and Donnie moves in, hunches, and sticks his eye into the eyepiece. "Oooooh, boys," he says. "There are *two* shooters in there. They probably bedded down high up on that hill overnight to avoid predators, and I'm thinking they're going to eat their way into and down the valley."

Donnie peels back and William moves in, dialing in the scope. "Oh yeah, definitely both shooters."

"Let me see those binoculars," I say to Donnie, who tosses me the pair.

William leads me to the caribou. "OK, you see that sort of black patch of rock at the middle bottom of the hill? Now walk up it until you see that section of light brown, then go right a bit . . . ," he says. I squint for about 30 seconds, until the white dots appear. "Got 'em," I say. There are perhaps 25 in the herd. Two stand out as burlier than the others—antlers wider, taller, and more meandrous.

"They don't seem to be moving downhill with any urgency," I say.

"Yeah, and they may even move back uphill," replies Donnie. From their current position they'll spot us and bolt if we try to move into the valley. So we'll sit, wait, and watch.

To kill time we start chatting about the ethics of technology in hunting. "Here we have this rifle that could easily shoot a caribou at five hundred yards or more," says Donnie. "But we're not going to do that. Because I don't think that's a fair chase. Some guys are even using rifles and tech to shoot a thousand yards. That's not hunting.

That's a video game. Those guys are so far away that even if the animal could see them it probably wouldn't consider them a threat."

Too little tech, on the other hand, can also be questionable. "You have people who are using longbows they made themselves and broadheads they carved from stone," says Donnie. "It's admirable. But those weapons are too low-tech and inefficient. They reduce the chance of a swift kill and often just injure the animal. What tool are you deadliest with, and how can you use that tool in a way that is on equal ground with the animal?" For Donnie the answer is somewhere between taking shots from multiple football fields away and shooting twigs with rocks attached to them.

He sees no real ethical difference between bows and rifles, so long as a person shoots close enough that the animal is more likely to catch you stalking in than not. "I prefer bows because they are silent," he says.

"Two deadheads down along the river," says William, referring to a pair of sun-bleached, antlered caribou skulls.

"That's a good sign," says Donnie. "Wolves and bears are hunting this area, too. It's more than likely that a lot of caribou move through here." Another hour passes.

I stand up and march in place. It's the only thing I can do to stay warm yet not attract animal attention. Another hour goes by.

"Herd's moving," says William.

Donnie rises and puts his eye to the scope. He watches for a half minute, then explains that the animals seem to be doing just as he expected: They're hoofing northward, low along the hill and down the valley.

The valley eventually climbs into a saddle that drops off into another wide valley. "If we can beat them to the other side of that saddle," Donnie says, "we'll be in a good position as they crest it. A very good position. But we have to move quick."

We frantically gather our gear then hunch and hike along the ridge. We're silent except for our labored breaths and the occasional pieces of shale crunching under our boots.

After 30 minutes of trekking we drop over the saddle into a rolling, wide-open valley. It smells like cedar, grass, and cold, clean water. The earth slopes nearly imperceptibly downward toward The Fort, a flat-topped shale butte that shoots 2,000 feet above the tundra with little run-up. Its sides are vertical cliffs. If it wasn't below freezing out and the rock was red instead of tan, chocolate, and gold, you could mistake the structure for something you'd find in the desert of southern Utah rather than the tundra of northern Alaska. Taller than they are wide, buttes are created by the work of water, wind, ice, and time. The Fort dominates the horizon, imposingly set in front of a blue sky with a few stratocumulus clouds guarding its flank.

Now out of the herd's sight, we can stand tall and crank. Donnie is like an army officer with a point to prove to his unfit men: hiking, hiking, hiking. Head glued forward and silently hiking us to our destination across the tundra, springs, and muck. I'm clambering across the land, trying my best to keep up without rolling an ankle on one of the godforsaken tussocks. We spook a flock of ptarmigan. They've shed their summer brown and transitioned to winter white. The gang brood swoops in sequence overhead, their white contrasting with the dull hills.

The same layers that 45 minutes ago weren't enough to keep the cold from chilling me to the core are now burning me up. There's no time to pause and strip them, so I open every zipper, welcoming the frigid Arctic air.

After 30 minutes of hiking Donnie stops, pulls his forearm and hand parallel to the ground, and with a flat palm pushes cold air toward the earth, signaling us to get down. "Stay here," he tells William and me. "I'm going to see if I can see them."

He tiptoes in the direction of where the herd would theoretically be if they followed the course we anticipated. As Donnie reaches the crest of a knoll he immediately spins backward. He's slamming his palm toward the ground and running all crouched. "They're coming over the saddle and moving directly toward us," he says as he reaches us.

He focuses on me. "I need you to listen and do everything I say."
I nod an OK.

"Get the rifle."

I unlash it from my bag as Donnie removes three 3.3-inch Hornady Outfitter 30-06 rifle cartridges from his pack and places them in a pocket. These rounds were built specifically for hunts in the most extreme conditions—their cases are watertight and designed to resist corrosion. He then explains that the caribou are now at our 11 o'clock and should walk right past us if we belly-crawl a couple hundred yards to our 7 o'clock.

Donnie dumps all but the down jacket and pants from his pack and slings it across his back. I cradle the rifle in my arms as I lie stomach-down in the dirt.

We army-crawl across the grass, shale, lichen, and twigs, shedding frost from the earth as we slide our hands and torsos along it. The only sounds are our breaths and rain jackets and canvas pants grating against the ground. Next we're in muck, its wet clay painting us. We crawl like this for roughly 100 yards. Then 200. Donnie stops. "Stay down," he says, slowly rising with the binoculars.

Nothing. We adjust course and cover another 100 yards.

Antlers appear at the apex of the saddle. They're like thick oak branches against the blue sky. It's a single set. Then there are two sets, then three and four. Then the faces and white muscular chests of the full herd appear, fog exiting their noses as they breathe and lumber toward us.

I've transitioned into a hunter, surveying the herd for its elders. But I didn't originally plan on hunting this place. As a journalist— someone who observes and reports rather than participates—I had reservations about getting too involved.

Donnie didn't push me. But he did tell me that by hunting I'd better understand our modern removal from the cycle of life. "Absolutely no pressure," he said. "It's an unbelievably big decision. But I do think you'd grasp why we're out here better if you were to hunt." I trusted him and became willing to cross what I presumed would be a heavy emotional barrier.

About 11.5 million Americans hunt, and a national poll conducted by scientists at Purdue University found that 87 percent of us find hunting acceptable, so long as the animal is being used for food. President Jimmy Carter, a lifelong hunter and fisherman, explaining his thoughts on the "uneasiness" one feels when killing an animal for food, wrote, "For people who might find these feelings overwhelming, my advice would be: 'Don't hunt or fish.' Indeed, if someone has a moral or ethical objection to taking an animal's life for human use, it is logical that he or she be a dedicated vegetarian and not require others, perhaps in a fish market or slaughterhouse, to end lives for their benefit; many make that decision."

The Purdue University researchers discovered that the people who viewed hunting favorably were more likely to have had interactions with livestock and live in rural areas. It was the people most removed from the food source—mostly urbanites who had experienced only perfectly manicured meat all lined up in earnest at the grocery store—who had the harshest opinion about killing one's own meat.

I'm also not against the responsible ownership of some guns. I own a couple. A 12-gauge pump action for shooting skeet and a 9mm handgun I purchased and took extensive training with after a drug addict attempted a forced entry into my home.

I've since found that shooting the handgun alone way out in the desert is its own paradoxical form of meditation. I get lost in the exercise of trying to relax and focus entirely on my breath as repeated explosions occur at the end of my hands.

But I didn't have much of a background in long-range shooting. So once I decided to hunt on this trip, I called a military sniper friend, who worked his network and looped me in with a local competitive rifleman and US marshal.

We met at a range in the Mojave Desert. He pulled two long cases from the bed of his F-150. We covered safety, body positioning, ballistics, and how to sight in objects and read weather patterns. After a long day in the desert I was dinging targets from 1,000 yards away.

"How far are you going to be shooting up there?" he asked me.

"Probably a little more than a hundred yards."

"If you can hit a target at a thousand yards," he said, "you'll be able to put the bullet on a quarter at a hundred yards."

Donnie pulls the three rounds from his pocket for me to place in the rifle's clip. I wait to cycle the bolt to shuttle a round into the chamber. I place the rifle on Donnie's pack, which forms a makeshift gun rest, and bring its butt into my right shoulder. Left hand on the forestock and right on the grip. As Donnie surveys the herd through binoculars I cock my head to peer through the scope.

They're strutting down the valley at our right flank. My arms, legs, and chest are filled with a nervy, high-frequency energy that feels like a million little pins dancing throughout my body.

"The two shooters are in there," says Donnie, breathing heavily. "The first is off to the left, and the second . . ." He pauses, then his intensity picks up. "The second is . . ."

He's there, bringing up the middle of the herd. I first notice his antlers. They're compact yet entirely complex—a freak piece of natural abstract art.

A flat shovel with minuscule points like a serrated blade bisects his face. A bez piece emerges from each antler base; they run at a 45-degree angle above his face and end in overpowering hands of flame. His main beams launch from his head and curve vertically like long wispy brushstrokes. As they rise, eight-inch conical back points shoot over his neck and back. After a few feet of travel the wispy main beams fork every which way, and each fork curvedly divides again and again, like long, demonic fingers. Fractals. The body behind the antlers is rotund and white in the chest and neck, clove brown in the torso.

His antlers hitch slightly to the left with each step. He's limping on a rear leg.

"That's your bull. The one that's limping," says Donnie. "He's old. Old. That's him. That's him."

A young bull comes too close. The old bull quickly jukes right, lowers his neck, and gores the young gun, a bully's warning to yield. As he moves he reveals a thick scar across his left hindquarter.

"Do you see him?!" Donnie whispers. "Do you see him?!"

"I see him," I say. My jugular vein is pulsing.

As the herd closes in I spin against the ground, keeping my body and the rifle's barrel a perfectly straight line pointed at the animals. The tundra's pillowy moss cushions my weight.

I occasionally catch him through the scope. When he appears I'll begin to anchor the crosshairs. Then he'll bob and weave between other caribou. His limp is a tell that makes each movement exaggerated and erratic. Just as he reappears, he falls back into the scrum.

"Do you see him now?!"

"No, I lost him in the herd."

I keep my eye in the scope and focus on my breathing. Three seconds in, five seconds out. Over and over, a sort of Zen in the art of ballistics.

The herd is but 100 yards from us now. "If you don't want to take the shot you shouldn't," says Donnie. "But if you're going to take the shot you need to take it soon."

They've moved past the closest point now. They're walking downwind from us and are extending the gap. They're at 110 yards, then 120 and 130. He's completely gone from the scope. I lift my eye from it, surveying the herd.

They're now 150 yards away. I return my eye to the scope and focus on the group where I last saw him. Two cows shift positions, creating a gap. I first see his antlers.

Then there he is. No animals within five feet. His head is down and he's eating. He stops. Raises his head to look down the horizon. Perhaps he caught our scent? I fill my lungs with air, then I begin to slowly release all that air back into the Arctic as I anchor the crosshairs just above his front shoulder.

17

12/31, 11:59:33 P.M.

I'D BEEN SOBER about 18 months and thought I was done with the big emotional swings. But then some stupid podcast I was listening to on my commute completely defeated me. The host was explaining a concept called the cosmic calendar. It puts all of time—the universe's 13.8 billion years—on a yearlong scale. So, in the cosmic calendar, the Big Bang occurred on January 1 at 12:00:00 a.m. The Milky Way galaxy formed on March 16. Our solar system took shape on September 2, and Earth followed on September 6, about 4.4 billion years ago. The first complex cells on Earth emerged on November 9. Dinosaurs appeared on Christmas and went extinct on December 30. And then the host said that on this calendar all of recorded human history—12,000 years and 480 generations of people—shows up on the night of December 31 at about 11:59 and 33 seconds.

When I heard that, I felt unfathomably insignificant in the grand scheme of time and space. I could see that I was going to die soon, and that all of the people I care about were also going to die soon. I realized that we'd all be forgotten soon after that. I could see there was nothing I could do about any of it. And I totally lost it.

But at that moment I was missing a higher reality. I didn't appreciate how lucky I was to be alive, and the miracle of being born in an age and place of health and prosperity. Instead I was bawling my eyes out in my V8-powered, air-conditioned, half-ton pickup that was streaming voices from outer freaking space.

One scientist calculated the numbers and found that a person's odds of being alive are 1 in 10 to the 2,685,000 power. The scientist explains that these odds are the same as having a group of 2 million people each roll a *trillion-sided* die and every roll landing on the same number. Like 550,343,279,007.

This figure also doesn't factor in my luck of being born in a developed country in recent time. Even about a century ago, for example, between 30 and 40 percent of European children died before turning 5. That's why in 1900 the average life expectancy in the world was 31. Now the world's average life expectancy is 72.

Yet as modern medicine, comforts, and conveniences have allowed humans more years, we've seemingly become less comfortable with death, life's only guarantee. Eight out of ten Westerners say they feel uncomfortable with death. Only half of people over 65 have considered how they want to die.

After someone dies we're encouraged to "stay busy" to "take our mind off it." A dead person's body is immediately covered and sent to a mortician, where it is either cremated and placed into a shiny new urn or prepared to look as youthful and alive as possible before one final, hourlong viewing, after which it is dropped into the ground of a perfectly manicured cemetery.

Ignoring death wasn't always the American way, said Gary Laderman, PhD, a death historian at Emory University. "In the nineteenth century and before, Americans were much more intimate with death and it was much more a part of everyday life—death was family and community based. It was homespun and homegrown. When someone died the corpse was right there.

"The key turning point is Abraham Lincoln's death and funeral. Lincoln becomes the most public figure ever to be embalmed, and the process is described in newspapers," Laderman told me. "Embalming then becomes mainstream and the funeral industry grows and expands. For some it's the way to keep death distant, a way to not see death or face it."

This coincided with "the rise of the modern hospital. Funerals and hospitals began to kind of take over the process of dying and the dead body," said Laderman. A sick person goes into the hospital, then to the funeral home, then into the ground—the process is off our hands. "Hospitals leveraged knowledge and expertise to bring death out of its former intimacy."

With the rise of medicine, we also began believing science would always save us, said Laderman. We now overmedicalize, undergoing more pain and suffering at the end of life for the possibility of delaying death. Harvard Medical School surgery professor and recipient of a MacArthur "Genius" grant Dr. Atul Gawande notes that 25 percent of all Medicare spending is for the 5 percent of patients in their final year of life. Most of that money goes to treatments that are of little lifesaving benefit and often just put the person through more unnecessary suffering.

We take weird supplements, believe impossible things, and undergo bizarre procedures to try to push death a few days downfield. In my career I've written about men who in the name of living longer have illegally acquired dangerous pharmaceuticals from overseas labs, paid thousands to have the blood of younger men pumped into their bodies, and spent millions funding teams of scientists who will, they believe, discover a fountain of youth in pill form.

Alternatively many of us are so unaware of our impending death that we forget to live true to ourselves, which is one of the most common regrets of Americans on their deathbeds. There is, indeed, a reason why people who encounter near-death experiences often quit their mundane jobs or end toxic relationships to pursue their dreams.

Existential philosopher Martin Heidegger said, "If I take death into my life, acknowledge it, and face it squarely, I will free myself from the anxiety of death and the pettiness of life—and only then will I be free to become myself."

Recently, scientists at the University of Kentucky tested whether there was any wisdom in those words. They had one group of people think about a painful visit to the dentist and the other contemplate their own death. The death thinkers afterward encountered a new-found perspective. They reported being more happy and fulfilled in life. The scientists concluded, "Death is a psychologically threatening fact, but when people contemplate it, apparently the automatic system begins to search for happy thoughts."

The country of Bhutan—which if people know it at all is probably because it often turns up second to Disneyland on lists of the "happiest places on earth"—has made it part of their national curriculum to think about death anywhere from one to three times daily. The understanding that we're all going to die is hammered into Bhutan's collective conscience. Death is part of everyday life. Ashes of the dead are mixed with clay and molded into small pyramids, called *tsha-tshas,* and placed in visible public areas—along heavily trafficked roadsides, on windowsills, and in public squares and parks. Bhutanese art often centers around death; paintings of vultures picking the flesh from corpses, dances that reenact dying. Funerals are a 21-day event where the dead body "lives" in its house before being slowly cremated over fragrant juniper trees in front of hundreds of friends and relatives.

All of this death is no buzzkill for the Bhutanese—quite the opposite. Despite being ranked 134 on the list of most-developed nations on earth, extensive studies conducted by Japanese researchers have found that Bhutan is among the world's 20 happiest countries. But what most people don't know is how the Bhutanese's morbid interest in death contributes to their feelings of happiness. And neither did I.

And so, after four flights across 48 hours, 14 time zones, and 9,465 miles, I stepped off an aging 737 onto a runway 7,333 feet above sea level at Bhutan's Paro International Airport. A thin air filled my lungs as the sun illuminated the surrounding foothills of the snow-capped Himalayas.

I'D ARRANGED FIRST TO MEET DASHO KARMA URA. THE IDEA THAT THINKING ABOUT death might have something to do with Bhutanese joy was compelling, but it also carried an aura of mysticism.

I wanted to start with hard numbers, facts, and figures. Those with a side of philosophy are exactly what Karma Ura delivers. Death-pondering isn't his primary job but is instead a by-product of leading the Centre for Bhutan & GNH [Gross National Happiness] Research, a government-backed social science research institute in Thimphu, Bhutan's capital. *Dasho* is a special Bhutanese title for a high-ranking government official. Like Secretary of (insert department, like "State," or "Defense," or "Health and Human Services").

The dasho is essentially Bhutan's Secretary of Happiness. He has for two decades studied happiness—what makes people happy and what a government can do to promote it. The *New York Times* recently referred to him as "one of the world's leading experts on happiness."

He conducts extensive happiness studies throughout the country and makes happiness policy recommendations to the royal government. It's a fitting job. The man is a serious quant. "Our data collected from over eight thousand randomly sampled Bhutanese above fifteen years old every four years consistently shows high national averages of satisfaction with life," he said. "Overall these put Bhutan among the top twenty in happiness rankings." One of his team's recent studies found that only 8.8 percent of Bhutanese say they're unhappy and the remaining 91.2 percent report being "narrowly," "extensively," or "deeply" happy.

In 1972, King Jigme Singye Wangchuck of Bhutan noticed that most countries strive to build a high gross domestic product. But in doing so they often create overworked middle and upper classes and a miserable lower class. What's more, the countries often have to destroy the environment in the hunt for resources and money, metrics that drive GDP.

The king told a reporter, "Gross National Happiness is more important than Gross National Product." He was espousing the idea that economic growth isn't an end in itself but rather a means to achieve a more important end, which is happiness. So why not just figure out what makes people happy and chase that?

The Bhutanese government then set out to improve in their country nine qualities that research shows breed happiness. Qualities like psychological well-being, physical health, ideal working standards, cultural diversity and resilience, strong community, ecological resilience, and adequate living standards.

Dorji, my driver (the law in Bhutan requires all tourists to hire both a guide and a driver), had brought me to the dasho's hillside home. We were sitting there with a hot woodstove between us. The dasho—minuscule, bespectacled, and erudite—was dressed in a plain dark *gho*. His voice was a slow whisper that I struggled to pick up over the embers popping from within the stove.

The dasho was part of a 1980s-era program that picked the brightest young people from highly underdeveloped nations and sent them for advanced degrees at Oxford University. That's where he studied economics and philosophy. Which explains his philosophical side, a side that seems to understand the shortcomings of numbers and how many aspects of the human experience cannot be measured.

"In the West you often see a reduction of measuring everything with money," he said as he leaned back, hands clasped over his stomach. "So many things are not, cannot, and should not be substituted by money and economic metrics."

His wife entered the room with mugs of *suja,* a traditional Bhutanese tea mixed with butter and salt. I told him about how, despite our massive GDP, the United States recently experienced an extended period where life expectancy dropped. He took a sip of tea, the steam fogging his glasses, then paused to think.

"The reduction of life expectancy is a very serious indicator that means there are many underlying factors that are undermining well-being," he said. "I think that external conditions may be improving in the United States."

He pointed out that our economy is strong and that we have many opportunities and creature comforts. "But the internal conditions in the United States may not be. Because well-being is really a by-product of the interaction between a person's external and internal conditions. And you can become very brittle and make fatalistic decisions without your internal conditions well maintained."

His work shows that happiness has less to do with external comforts than many Westerners think. And Western scholars agree. Researchers at Stanford noted, "An extraordinary finding that's been replicated over and over is that once you get past the 25 percent or so poorest countries on earth, where the only question is survival and subsistence, there is no relationship between gross national product, per capita income, any of those things, and levels of happiness."

Bhutan lags far behind in the financial department. The average person in Bhutan earns just $225 a month. The International Monetary Fund ranks the country 161 of 185 in gross domestic product, a measure of all the stuff a country produces. Many of the country's roads aren't paved. Thimphu is the only capital city in the world without a stoplight. As of 2017 less than half the country had Internet access. There is no McDonald's, Burger King, or Starbucks.

I asked him why most Bhutanese seem to be so happy, despite the nation not ranking highly in development.

"There are likely many reasons for this," he said. "We have deep community connections here, but also deep connections to the landscape." Roughly 70 percent of the Bhutanese live in rural areas, in small communities of about 200 people (recall the Savanna Theory of Happiness). Most people own land.

"This landscape . . . the same mountain slope . . . it is a person's birthplace, their workplace, their growth place, and it is their death place. So in that sense they might feel a sense of belonging to a community and familiar landscape," said the dasho. "This wider idea of seeing yourself as embedded to a place is probably not there in America. People move so often and mostly live in cities. Belonging is probably more abstract, like belonging to brands like Nike or something." Fast Company recently reported that more big American corporations are dumping money into building a sense of "brand belonging," a sort of advertorial shift from "buy us" to "be us."

The dasho's surveys discovered that the Bhutanese rank mental and physical health as the most important source of happiness. The obesity rate in Bhutan is just 6 percent. "Bhutan's medical healthcare provisions are not great," he said. "But they are free. Every procedure is paid for by the government. And if the hospitals here cannot perform a procedure well enough, then they will cover all expenses to do the procedure outside Bhutan."

Which leads the dasho to his next point: "The Bhutanese also have less debt," he said. "All Bhutanese own their own house. Americans don't. Maybe the quality of the Bhutanese houses isn't as good. But they have windows looking across the valley and the forest in the back. The sense of freedom you experience not being tied to debt is significant."

The dasho is seeing that the influence of mobile tech is causing more young Bhutanese to migrate into cities like Thimphu and Paro. But even these "cities" are what we in America might consider cute mountain ski towns, and their citizens essentially live and work in nature.

"We know access to nature is fundamental," he continued. "It engages all five senses, and you have to experience it daily to be impacted by it. It can help you see yourself through a different perspective. Maybe you see a wild boar in the forest and wonder what his existence is like, and you realize his life is so much more of a struggle. And nature has both a beauty and a mortality to it. You see the cycles it goes through and it reminds you that you yourself are going through cycles."

It felt like the right moment to transition to the reason for my trip. I asked him how he believes the Bhutanese relationship with death factors into happiness.

"Death cannot just be a matter of hospitals and funeral homes and insurance and money transactions," he said. "You need some sort of pedagogy. In Bhutan we learn that to see yourself as not always a living person, but also a dying person, is a very important pedagogy of life. Death here is part of the culture and communication."

It's difficult to measure exactly how the country's death consciousness improves happiness. His surveys do, however, measure spirituality. He said death is baked into the foundation of Buddhism, the country's main faith. And the Bhutanese brand of Buddhism seems to put more emphasis on being aware of death than most other primarily Buddhist nations. But, he said, he'll leave the deeper theological death lessons to the man I'm meeting next.

I LOADED BACK INTO DORJI'S SUPERCOMPACT HATCHBACK. DORJI WAS WEARING A traditional Bhutanese gho and chewing *rajnigandha,* which is areca nut shell and betel leaf coated in a flavor that tastes like burning incense. He drove us thirty minutes down a paved highway, then dodged a pack of five stray dogs as he turned onto a steep dirt road. The car's tires ricocheted off the rocky road. We sent up dust as we passed kids playing in front of traditional wooden houses, a row of Buddhist prayer wheels, and a group of aged women walking uphill with bales of hay strapped to their backs.

The road worsened with the altitude. Dorji was traversing a 4x4 trail in what was essentially a smart car with a backseat. We were thrown all about as he madly cranked the wheel and liberally throttled the engine, forcing the car to crawl over bumps. The car's frame produced a deep grinding noise as it scraped against uneven earth. The road rose and twisted past tiered rice fields and cliffs.

After 30 minutes of Baja-500-esque driving, we pulled to the side of the road. "Two hours," I said, holding up two fingers. Dorji smiled and nodded. Killed the engine, pulled the emergency brake, rolled down the windows, and fully reclined his seat. A cool wind shook the needles of the surrounding pines as I began the ten-minute hike along a cliffside trail. Now that I'd heard the statistics, it was time to speak with the mystics.

The first was Khenpo Phuntsho Tashi. He knows as much about death as a living human can. He's one of Bhutan's leading Buddhist thinkers, and he's found a niche in the study of death and dying. The *khenpo* is the author of a 250-page book called *The Fine Art of Living and Manifesting a Peaceful Death.* And, unlike many of Bhutan's monks, the khenpo is intimately familiar with what ails people in the West. Before he dedicated himself to his spiritual practice, he lived in Atlanta with a girlfriend who was the Dalai Lama's translator. He, I thought, would be able to get to the heart and consequences of the West's fear of death.

My boots kicked up a low-hanging dust as the khenpo's cliffside shack came into view. It was wooden, tin roofed, and in the shadow of Dakarpo, an ancient Buddhist monastery built on an outcropping overlooking the Shaba valley. Fifteen or so people walked clockwise around the white, fortress-like monastery. They chanted as they carefully stepped along its rocky terrain. Bhutanese mythology says a person will be cleared of all of his or her sins by circumnavigating the Dakarpo 108 times. Each lap takes roughly 25 minutes. Completing the full 108 turns takes most pilgrims about four days, a relatively small fee for absolute absolution.

A woman greeted me at the door of the shack. She pointed to a cast-iron bucket filled with sand, out of which stuck a few burning incense sticks. I wafted their smoke into my face. She then took a golden kettle imprinted with Sanskrit and poured water into my hands. I drank half and placed the rest atop my head. Now purified, I removed my boots and stepped into the shack.

Its first room was bare except for a tabby cat curled up on a meditation cushion. My footsteps creaked the floorboards as I stepped into the next room, which was a simple kitchen with basic tools for cooking—knives, bowls, and an electric cooktop. To the right was one last draped doorway.

The scent of burning incense crawled into my nose as I peeled back the heavy, embroidered orange silk drape. Light was entering the room through a hazy window, illuminating smoke. It obscured a small altar anchored by a three-foot statue of the Buddha. Around it were smaller Buddhist statues, photographs, and burning sticks of *champa*. Through the smoke I saw the profile of a face. It was the khenpo.

Dressed in maroon-and-gold robes, he was sitting in a meditative lotus position on an ornate cushion atop a small platform. He slowly turned his head and smiled as we locked eyes. If I'd had any preconceived notions about what kind of scene I'd be walking into after traveling to a real-life Shangri-La to consult a leading monk in his cliffside monastery shack, this scene was . . . well . . . exactly what I'd pictured. Looking at him, I couldn't help but think of Bill Murray as groundskeeper Carl Spackler in *Caddyshack* describing the Dalai Lama: "The flowing robes . . . the grace . . . bald . . . striking."

"Welcome," said the khenpo, his voice a heavily accented butter. I bowed and sat. "You want to talk about death?"

I nodded. "Hmmmm," he said. His chest slowly rose and fell in the silence.

"You Americans are usually ignorant," he said, using a word that is often seen as an insult in the United States but that by definition means "lacking awareness." In Bhutan and other Buddhist countries, "ignorance" is the rough English translation of *Avidyā*, a Sanskrit word that means having a misunderstanding of the true nature of your reality and the truth of your impermanence. "Most Americans are unaware of how good you have it, and so, many of you are miserable and chasing the wrong things," he said.

"What are these wrong things?" I asked, looking for the pose and tone one should take when speaking to a religious authority.

"You act like life is fulfilling a checklist. 'I need to get a good wife or husband, then I get a good car, then I get a good house, then I get a promotion, then I get a better car and a better house and I make a name for myself and then . . .'" He rattled off more accomplishments that fulfill the American Dream. "But this plan will never materialize perfectly. And even if it does, then what? You don't settle, you add more items to the checklist. It is the nature of desire to get one thing and immediately want the next thing, and this cycle of accomplishment and acquisitions won't necessarily make you happy—if you have ten pairs of shoes you want eleven pairs."

He's not wrong. Stuff collection has increased in the United States over the last 100 years. The average American woman in the 1930s, for example, had 36 clothing items in her closet. People today who consulted a decluttering service were found to have 120, and most of them were rarely worn. According to scientists at the University of California–Riverside, material goods fall prey to a similar "creep" phenomenon. They give us a burst of cheer. That is, until we've had them for a moment, which is when we lose interest and the next material desire consumes our mind.

Researchers at San Francisco State University found that titles, wealth, and possessions ultimately improve our well-being only insofar as they fulfill our basic needs. For example, having enough money to buy a safe home, sufficient food, and a car that works might increase our happiness. But there isn't much long-term difference in the well-being one gets from, say, living in a modest home versus a McMansion or commuting in a base-model Mazda versus a Maserati. The researchers, in fact, found a paradox: being overly materialistic leads to unhappiness.

Perhaps this is why minimalism and the "life-changing magic" of getting rid of stuff is now popular in America. It all seems good in theory. But some scholars have argued that American attempts to dematerialize are just another form of materialism. As University of Iowa anthropologist Meena Khandelwal put it, we now simplify not because we're "surrendering ourselves to some higher reality," like the khenpo, but rather because minimalism looks good on Instagram.

The khenpo then pointed out that by blindly pursuing this check-list, we're often forced into acts that take us away from that higher re-ality and happiness. He was echoing a sentiment shared among many leaders in the tradition of Vajrayana Buddhism. Sogral Rinpoche, in his 1992 work *The Tibetan Book of Living and Dying,* calls this check-list phenomenon "Western laziness." It consists of "cramming our lives with compulsive activity, so that there is no time at all to confront the real issues. . . . If we look into our lives, we will see clearly how many unimportant tasks, so-called 'responsibilities' accumulate to fill them up. . . . Going on as we do, obsessively trying to improve our condi-tions, can become an end in itself and a pointless distraction."

The average American works 47 hours a week. Our entrepreneurs and "productivity gurus" preach that a "grind" and "shut up and work harder" mentality is the secret to satisfaction. American busyness has radically increased since the 1960s, and scientists at the Columbia Business School in a series of studies showed that we increasingly see busyness as a way to earn status. This mentality may be a mod-ern substitute filling a void left when we stopped doing physically difficult things. For example, Elon Musk boasts about working 120 hours a week, and Chris Cuomo referred to himself as a "warrior" for working through his bout with the coronavirus.

This upset in our work-life balance—or, perhaps, our problem integrating our work into our life and not the other way around—factors into why other research has shown that America is, in fact, less happy than it was decades ago.

"So this checklist plan does not make you truly happy. Then what?" said the khenpo. He was silent. Left it open for me to ponder.

"I don't know. I'm an ignorant American," I said, and smiled.

"Then you could be happier!" he responded with a chuckle. "Whereas if you understand this cycle and nature of mind and you prioritize mindfulness, then everything will be OK. Even if you don't become rich. Fine, you're mindful. Even if you don't get a perfect wife? Fine, you're mindful."

Ah, yes. "Mindfulness." That squishy, what-the-hell-does-that-even-mean word that's so hot in America today but has, in fact, been a part of Eastern traditions since before Christ. It's roughly defined as purposefully paying attention to what's happening in the present moment without judgment, according to Jon Kabat Zinn, a professor at the University of Massachusetts Medical School and pioneer of mindfulness in the Western world. In other words, it's being aware of what's going on upstairs.

Being about as enlightened as the floorboards I sat on in the khenpo's shack, I've had trouble with mindfulness. I've meditated every day in sobriety. I flounder most of the time, but the practice usually downgrades my mind from a category 5 hurricane to a category 4. This gives me fleeting moments where I can see the mental machinery for what it really is. Which feels like progress.

But the khenpo made mindfulness sound akin to jamming a stick into the spokes of the checklist and developing a state of okayness. In other words, whether I'm rich or poor or famous or a nobody, I should avoid becoming caught up in the narratives my mind spits out and just accept the direction of things. This will help me go beyond the checklist and be just fine.

This brand of thinking, it occurred to me, is in some ways what's kept me sober. Any time something bad happened to me I'd just remind myself that things would be that much worse if I were still on the sauce.

The woman who had taken me through the cleansing ritual entered the room. She placed a plate of cucumbers and mandarin orange wedges on the floor between the khenpo and me. "All organic!" he said, and grabbed a spear of cucumber. It crunched as he bit into it.

"OK, then how do you get a Westerner like me, who has been conditioned to achieve the checklist, to live more mindfully?" I asked.

"Well, the Bhutanese, we also have ignorance, anger, and attachment. We have the same problems of the checklist. But, I think, less. This is because we apply what we call mindfulness of the body. We remember that everyone is dying right now," said the khenpo. "Everyone will die. You are not singled out. Do you *know* this? To not think of death and not prepare for it . . . this is the root of ignorance."

Pretend you are walking along a trail, he explained, and there is a cliff in 500 yards. The catch—the cliff is death, we will all walk off it, and we are, in fact, walking toward it this very moment. "Buddha died. Jesus died. You will die. I will die. I would like to die on that bed," said the khenpo, pointing to a twin mattress on the floor.

"Don't you want to know that there's a cliff?" he asked. Because only then can we change our course. We could take a more scenic route, notice the beauty of the trail before it ends, say the things we truly want to say to the people we're walking it with.

"When you start to understand that death is coming, that the cliff is coming, you see things differently. You change your mental course—you naturally become more compassionate and mindful," said the khenpo. "But Americans, they don't want to hear about the cliff. They don't think about death. After a funeral they want to get their mind off the death and just eat cake. The Bhutanese, they want to know about the cliff and they will be happy to talk about death and ruin the cake-eating.

"So remember," he continued, able to sustain the perfect upright lotus position while I was slumping and couldn't feel my legs, "we are all dying right now. To develop this mindfulness of death you have to think of *mitakpa*."

"Mitakpa?" I asked.

"Yes," he said. "Mitakpa."

Before I could probe the khenpo on what mitakpa is and what it might be able to do, my time was up and I was back in Dorji's hatchback. We were like bouncy balls in the seats as gravity aggressively pulled the car over all the rocks and ruts that once held us back. As we descended I asked, "Dorji, what is 'mitakpa'?" He looked at me and shook his head. "Mi-tak-pa," I said.

"Oh. *Mitakpa*," he replied, pronouncing the word less like an ignorant American. "Takpa, 'permanent,'" he said. "Mi, 'no.' Mitakpa, 'no permanent.'"

I began to ask him to explain further, but a Bhutanese traffic jam interrupted me. A herd of seven bulls and cows ambled up the one-lane road. Dorji pressed into the brake to slow the car to a crawl. The half-ton animals lazily parted around us, their bells clanking as they slid along the length of the hatchback.

He dropped me at my hotel. I was planning to cram in some work before dinner. Checklist stuff. But my conversation with the khenpo was high in my mind, so I instead decided to walk out into Thimphu. Passing rows of shops, I thought about death and my own relationship with the checklist.

I've experienced that "creep" phenomenon often. Like when a raise that I thought would radically improve my happiness gave me just a fleeting hit of joy. Or when I thought a purchase might change how people would view me and, therefore, make me happier. But in pursuit of sobriety I realized there are roughly five creatures who deeply care about me. Two of them are dogs. And all of them care about me for reasons that have nothing to do with my spending habits.

The public intellectual, philosopher, and neuroscientist Sam Harris writes that the checklist phenomenon is ultimately driven by our search to "finally relax and enjoy in the present." But we generally don't understand the underlying purpose of this search. And so we chase the checklist for the sake of it, which is "a false hope," he writes.

The lasting shifts in happiness I've experienced haven't come from anything societally imposed. Not money, degrees, titles, jobs, stuff. They've come from shifts in my mental state. Like after I got sober and could better do right by others. Or when I understood that I'm not that damn important, established a relationship with a power greater than myself, and realized that this power, as West Texas poet Terry Allen put it, "ain't somewhere up in the air, it's sittin' right here inside with you." The understanding that happiness is, yeah, sittin' right here inside of me, I guess, is a form of mindfulness.

A shaggy white dog singled me out and jumped up on my leg. He must have been hungry. I walked into a market stall that was selling baked goods and bought way too many sel roti, a type of Bhutanese doughnut. "No one owns the dogs," Dorji told me. "We all take care of them." For the rest of the night I walked around Thimphu feeding strays.

DORJI WAS BACK AT 9 A.M. HE DROVE US INTO THIMPHU'S DOWNTOWN AND THROUGH its one "stoplight," which is a police officer artfully directing traffic in the middle of a roundabout. We parked along the street, beneath a three-story apartment building.

I was here to meet Lama Damcho Gyeltshen. He doesn't ponder death in any abstract sense—he experiences it every day. He's the head lama at the Jigme Dorji Wangchuck National Referral Hospital, the main hospital in Bhutan. There he counsels the dying. After the khenpo elucidated the problem and hinted at some solution, the lama, I figured, might be able to expand.

Jigme Thinley was waiting for me as I stepped out of the car. He's a sort of do-everything for Dasho Karma Ura. The dasho thought it would be wise for me to meet with the lama and sent Jigme along to help bridge the language gap. Jigme was wearing a full gho. Wide, chiseled face and stout overbuilt frame. If it weren't for his nerdy wire glasses, he'd look better suited for farm labor or Division I wrestling than intellectual desk work.

Jigme and I climbed the apartment building's open-air concrete steps to its second floor. A dirty dog was curled up on a welcome mat. Jigme knocked and we were led into a sitting room where a handful of women cheerfully gabbed in Bhutanese. Shoes lined the entrance, their backs flattened like makeshift clogs. The Bhutanese have perfected the art of removing shoes, which is a requirement for entering homes and places of worship. I was in leather work boots with complicated laces. Everyone watched and giggled as I bent over and arduously unlaced and pulled off the clunky boots. "Not wise shoes for Bhutan," said Jigme with a smile.

We headed into the next room. The lama was sitting on a platform that was covered in silk meditation pads. He hopped off it as we entered. He and I shook hands and did a lot of smiling and nodding. He was bald, short, and doughy, with wire-framed glasses. His bright white smile popped against his blaze-orange robes. He sat back atop the platform, in the lotus, while Jigme and I sat on the floor. Jigme explained what I was there to talk about. Death, dying, and the Bhutanese death complex.

"Well, first I'd like to thank you for coming and reminding me of death, because it is important for the mind," said the lama. His words, naturally, set me up to ask why.

"When people come into my hospital there is a chance they leave," he said. "But there is also a high chance they do not leave. My job is to help people prepare for death. I have found that the people who have not thought about death are the ones who have regrets on their deathbeds, because they have not used a necessary tool that could have made them live a fuller life." An American study conducted across various hospitals like the Yale Cancer Center, Dana-Farber Cancer Institute, and Massachusetts General Hospital supports this notion. It found that dying patients who had open conversations about their death experienced a better quality of life in the weeks and months leading to their passing, as judged by their family members and nurse practitioners.

"The mind is afflicted with many delusions. But they come down to three," continued the lama. "And those are greed, anger, and ignorance. When your mind is not taken care of, these three things have an advantage. The dying people I counsel . . . they suddenly do not care about getting famous, or their car or watch, or working more. They don't care about the things that once angered them." In other words: When a person realizes death is imminent, their checklist and everyday bullshit becomes irrelevant and their mind begins to center on that which makes it happy. Research from Australia found that the top regrets of the dying include not living in the moment, working too often, and living a life the person thinks they should rather than one they truly want to.

"Whereas those who have thought of their death and prepared for it," said the lama, "they do not have those regrets. Because they have often not fallen so much into those delusions. They have lived in the moment. Maybe they have accomplished a lot, maybe they have not. But regardless it has not affected their happiness as much. . . ." He expanded on this phenomenon, explaining that a sort of cosmic psychic shift often occurs in the dying, bringing them closer to the things that matter in the end. A living person who thinks of dying will, yes, initially face mental discomfort, but they'll emerge on the other side having stolen a bit of this end-of-life magic.

"What is mitakpa?" I asked. "Someone told me it translates to 'no permanent.'"

"Close. Mitakpa is 'impermanence,'" said the lama. He raised an arm and finger, like a professor stressing a point. "Impermanence, impermanence, impermanence." This, he said, is the cornerstone of Buddhist teachings. It's the idea that everything is, well, impermanent. Nothing lasts and, therefore, nothing can be held on to.* By trying to hold on to that which is changing, like our life itself, we ultimately end up suffering. The Buddha's final words were on impermanence,

* The Buddhists, in fact, were death conscious hundreds of years before the Stoics.

a reminder that all things die. "All things change. Whatever is born is subject to decay . . . ," he said. "All individual things pass away."

As the cosmic calendar runs on, even our planet will die. Scientists have theorized a handful of ways Earth could be destroyed in the next billion or so years—asteroids, the sun becoming hotter as it burns out, etc. The entire universe itself may experience demise. The Big Rip theory suggests that a peculiar force called dark energy will eventually shred all of the universe's 10 to the 80th power atoms in a spectacular, all-encompassing intergalactic self-immolation.

"It's important to preserve this precious understanding of mitakpa in your mind. It will significantly contribute to your happiness," said the lama. He echoed the khenpo's sentiment, explaining that ignoring mitakpa often leads a person to believe that "things will be better when I do *x*." A false sense of permanence can cause a person to put off the things they truly want to do, thinking, "I can do that when I retire."

"But when you understand that nothing is permanent you cannot help but follow a better, happier path," he said. "It calms your mind. You tend not to get overly excited, angry, or critical. With this principle people interact with others and it improves their relationships. They become more grateful and gratuitous. Because they realize all their material goods and status will not matter in the end." And not just in Bhutan. A study in *Psychological Science* discovered that people who thought about their own death were more likely to show concern for people around them. They did things like donate time, money, and their own blood to blood banks.

It works on even the most hardened among us. Another study found that when American and Iranian religious fundamentalists were told to think about death they became more peaceful and compassionate toward opposition groups.

A team of researchers at Eastern Washington University found that thinking about death enhances gratitude. The scientists wrote that when people think about death they "tend to recognize 'what might not be' and become more grateful for the life they now experience. Fully recognizing one's own mortality may be an important aspect of the humble and grateful person. Perhaps when we recognize that death is a reality we all must face, we may then realize . . . that 'Life is not only a pleasure but a kind of eccentric privilege'" (as turn-of-the-century writer G. K. Chesterton put it). Gratitude has been shown to reduce anxiety and even ailments like heart disease.

"How often should I be thinking about mitakpa?" I asked.

"You must think of mitakpa three times each day. Once in the morning, once in the afternoon, and once in the evening. You must be curious about your death. You must understand that you don't know how you will die or where you will die. Just that you will die. And that death can come at any time," he said. "The ancient monks would remind themselves of this every time they left their meditation cave. I, too, remind myself of this every time I walk out my front door."

We talked for a half hour more about death and his work at the hospital. Then it was time for me to leave.

"Remember," said the lama as we were saying goodbye, "death can come at any time. Any time."

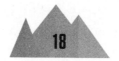

20 MINUTES, 11 SECONDS

I PULL THE rifle's trigger, an action that sends its striker pin into the round's primer, igniting the powder and creating a violent release of energy that pushes a bullet 22 inches down the barrel at 1,772 miles an hour.

The herd collectively flinches as pressure releases from the gun, interrupting the Arctic silence. They all freeze and survey in different directions. The old bull is nonreactive.

"Did you hit him?!"

"I don't know," I say. "I don't know." I forcefully pull back the bolt, ejecting the spent cartridge.

"I think you did. Shoot again. Shoot again," Donnie says.

Once that first bullet connects, a hunter is all in. There's no waiting to see if the shot was deadly. Just send more bullets. Because each second is another sliver of time the animal might suffer.

I firmly push the bolt back into position. This cycles another round into the chamber. Then I'm again searching the crosshairs for the bull's front shoulder. I fix on the target, exhale, and pull the trigger, restarting the ballistic process. The rifle's boom is immediately followed by a sharp *thwap*. I pull my eye from the scope.

The second shot causes all but one of the herd to sprint for higher ground. They are just like humans in a similarly dangerous situation. The first boom incites quizzical, nervous looks. The second sends us running.

The old bull remains. Then he falls out of sight. I pull the scope to my eye, but I can't see him. *Oh, God, what have I done?* I think as I stand and march toward him.

I first see one of his legs spastically kicking. I start running, rifle in hand. "Whoa, whoa," says Donnie, trailing behind me. "Slow down. He's dead. That movement is natural." The phenomenon applies to recently expired humans, too, and is caused by the nervous system spilling stored energy.

His antlers and clove-brown-and-white body come into full view. He's lying on his side on the mossy green tundra, like a sleeping horse. I stop about ten feet from him. "William and I will go back and get our gear," says Donnie.

Blood is falling a drop per second from the caribou's neck. It leaves a thin red stream through his heavy white mane, which is quaking in the cool Arctic breeze. I'd think he was resting were it not for that tiniest bit of evidence.

His thick body holds stories. The big scar on his back leg. Hooves worn from hundreds of thousands of miles of roaming this landscape. Teeth masticated into flat dishes from so many days of eating plants. His antlers spike and swoop and shovel and turn and thrust their way from his head. What kind of fights have they seen? His coat is thick and dense. What kind of storms has it weathered?

I sit next to him, place my hand on his head, and look out across the tundra. The land falls away, ramps up to The Fort, then lumbers 100 some-odd miles down into wide shale canyons and piney open valleys to the Chukchi Sea. His herd is now grazing the hill from which they came.

Conflicting emotions of sadness and elation rise within me. My body is heavy yet pulsing with energy. It is a feeling of intense closeness to and gratitude for this animal and the place from which he came. Almost like love.

Jim Posewitz, biologist, ethicist, and hunter, wrote in *Beyond Fair Chase: The Ethic and Tradition of Hunting,* "Hunting is one of the last ways we have to exercise our passion to belong to the earth, to be part of the natural world, to participate in the ecological drama, and to nurture the ember of wilderness within ourselves." I understand the sentiment, but it also comes with a heavy and burdensome emotional buy-in. I'm no longer a tourist here. I'm a participant.

This pursuit of holistically connecting to nature—mind, body, spirit—through hunting is likely why backcountry hunting has grown over the past decade. That's according to Land Tawney, the president of Backcountry Hunters and Anglers, a conservation group that fights to maintain public access to wild American lands. Their membership jumped from 1,000 in 2014 to more than 40,000 as of early 2020. I'd met with Tawney in Las Vegas before heading into the Arctic. He told me, "The idea of killing your own meat. Working hard for it and knowing where it's from. Hunting will surely teach you that, and make you thankful for *all* meat."

A squawk rockets me into the now. A raven is circling overhead, waiting for his dinner of caribou entrails.

Donnie and William are back. "That's a beautiful bull," says Donnie. "Spectacular. Absolutely spectacular."

William drops to his knees behind the caribou's neck and runs his hands over the antlers. "These back points are awesome," he says. "You don't see them this long. So unique."

"This bull wouldn't score much in antler record books, but he's as handsome as the day is long," says Donnie. "And he has a long history in the wild." We stand together and quietly admire him.

"Let's get to work," says William. He pulls a knife from his pack, unsheathes it, and sharpens it on a soapstone stored in the knife's case. Donnie removes his own knife and flicks his finger across its blade.

We all kneel around the caribou and as a team flip him onto his back. I hold the animal in place as William runs the blade down his midline, from pelvis to jaw. He accidentally punctures the stomach, leaving a quarter-inch cut that emits a hissing sound of exiting air. The knife continues its steadfast slide, reaching the breastbone, neck, then jaw.

Donnie, meanwhile, has cut a circle around the ankle of the caribou's left front leg, slicing through the tendon that connects the hoof. He twists off the hoof, then continues a long slice up the inside of the leg and peels back the skin. He then repeats the process on the back leg.

We ease the animal down onto his left side and peel back half the hide, resting it on the tundra like a rug. I stabilize the animal as William opens his chest cavity, revealing his entrails. Liver, kidneys, intestines, stomach. "We leave this open so wolverines, ravens, and other animals have easier access," Donnie says.

William reaches into the rib cage, sends another hand in with the knife, and emerges with the heart. It looks just like a human heart, only larger. Donnie and William inspect it.

"Your first shot hit him in the neck, in the carotid artery. But your second shot," says Donnie, holding up the organ like Hamlet while pointing to its bottom, "severed both ventricles of his heart. That killed him instantly. We'll eat this later."

"It's delicious," says William.

Steam rises from the animal's exposed muscle, which is smooth, fatless, and crimson. I pull his front leg upward. This gives Donnie space to cut through the connective tissue of the shoulder. The joint pops and the 35-pound front quarter swings free. I place it next to the heart on a tarp we've laid out.

"Here, take this, too," says William. It's a long tube of red meat that runs the length of the animal's back, called the backstrap in Cervidae and ribeye in cows.

Donnie and I transition to the back leg. I wasn't sure if the butchering process would make me cringe. But I'm grounded. My heart is still heavy, but as we break this caribou down I'm beginning to see a giver of meat and, therefore, life. This realization has forced me into something of an epiphany: I interact with dead animals by eating meat nearly every day. And not once have I shed a tear or felt much emotion when I leverage their flesh for my own needs. So I wonder: Why don't I feel this way about all the other meat I eat?

Charles List, PhD, a professor of philosophy at Plattsburgh State University of New York, said about our evolution from being hunters, "Our ancestors hunted because they absolutely had to. Modern hunting is a reenactment of that, but it ties into something deep inside us, because man evolved in a climate and culture of hunting and gathering. Because of this, hunting can change and move us in ways we wouldn't expect."

I pull the leg high so Donnie can again slide his blade along the connective tissue. The hindquarter—filled with sirloin, rump roast, bottom round, and eye of round—detaches, and I place it on the tarp. William works his knife from the top of the caribou's neck to its windpipe, then pulls off a cut of slightly fattier meat. He hands it to me to place on the tarp. "Because of the fat, the neck is great for burger meat," he says.

More meat comes my way, from Donnie. "This is the tenderloin," he says. "A lot of people don't know this is here, but it's some of the best meat on the caribou."

With the left side butchered, we carefully flip the caribou onto his right side and continue the work. Donnie pauses. "You doing all right?" he asks.

I tell him that I'm not entirely sure.

"It's heavy every single time," he says. "If it's ever not, then I'll stop hunting."

Thoreau saw hunting and its requisite emotions as necessary human education. In *Walden* he wrote: "Fishermen, hunters, woodchoppers, and others, spending their lives in the fields and woods, in a peculiar sense a part of Nature themselves, are often in a more favorable mood for observing her, in the intervals of their pursuits, than philosophers or poets even, who approach her with expectation."

Yet Thoreau was also aware of the great responsibility embedded in hunting. Again in *Walden* he wrote that it must be done "in earnest." He gave no definition of "in earnest." But Edward Abbey later interpreted Thoreau's "in earnest" to mean "done in a spirit of respect, reverence, gratitude."

As we work, Donnie begins to tell me that he often reminds himself that caribou don't age out, lying down to peacefully die on a bed of soft moss while surrounded by family. For one, caribou don't live in family units—they move in and out of herds, and caribou don't likely, according to research in *Current Biology,* experience grief. For another, their deaths are usually violent. "There are a handful of ways a caribou dies out here," says Donnie.

"The first is by predator," Donnie says as he works his blade around the right front ankle. "A grizzly bear or pack of wolves would have seen him with that limp and tried to take advantage. He'd be eaten alive over the course of twenty or so minutes.

"Then there's starvation. When caribou get old like this guy," he says, "they can't store fat as well. As the snow piles on everything, it would be harder for him to find enough quality food. Or his teeth get too worn down to chew. For caribou it's every animal for himself, and there is no helping an injured or hungry bull."

Donnie moves to the rear leg as I place the front quarter on the tarp. "They can also drown or freeze to death. Every year during migration the caribou cross a massive river system filled with ice. It's particularly dangerous for the youngest, oldest, and injured animals.

"Finally, there's competition. The males often fight each other. Sometimes to the death," he says. "Hold that leg, it's about to come off." He makes another cut and the final limb swings free.

"Did you see your bull gore that other one as they were coming over the hill? He's trying to maintain dominance. But eventually a younger, stronger bull will want to take that from him. They often get deeply gored and bleed out or become so injured that they slowly die."

We pause and watch William work the rest of the neck and head. "So when you consider all that," Donnie says, "I personally would take a 30-06 bullet to the heart and be dead in seconds. I'm anthropomorphizing here. But I think we can agree the bullet leads to less time suffering compared to the other options. Disney movies have led people to believe that nature is this harmonious place. It's not. Nature can be brutal." Philosophers call this flawed-but-common thinking the "appeal to nature" fallacy. It's the belief, argument, or rhetorical tactic that proposes that anything "natural" is good, harmonious, and morally correct.

President Teddy Roosevelt put it this way: "Death by violence, death by cold, death by starvation—these are the normal endings of the stately and beautiful creatures of the wilderness. The sentimentalists who prattle about the peaceful life of nature do not realize its utter mercilessness; . . . life is hard and cruel for all the lower creatures, and for man also in what the sentimentalists call a 'state of nature.'" The state humans lived in for all but the most recent fragment of time.

After two hours, all that remains of this caribou is the meat on the tarp, his antlered head sitting atop his cape, and his fat- and flesh-covered spinal column and intestines on the tundra.

A FEW DAYS AFTER I MET WITH THE LAMA IN BHUTAN, I CAME FACE-TO-FACE WITH his teachings. I'd spent the morning hiking five steep miles to Paro Taksang, The Tiger's Nest, a sacred 15th-century Buddhist monastery built in the traditional Bhutanese *dzong* style. The monastery sits at 10,240 feet above sea level and clings to a cliff like a reptile on a vertical wall. It's the location where in the eighth century, Padmasambhava, a man considered to be the "Second Buddha," meditated in a tiger-filled cave for three years, three months, three weeks, three days, and three hours.

I'd come to see the monastery's famous artwork, much of which depicts death. It holds various images and statues of, for example, Mahakala, a protector god whose crown is ringed with skulls and whose sash is strung with severed heads. His Sanskrit name translates to "beyond time" or, more simply, "death."

As I exited the monastery and put my shoes back on, Dorji hurriedly approached me. "Someone sick," he said in his broken English. He pointed up the trail, to a set of steep stairs cut from a cliff that led up to a small meditation hut next to a waterfall. Toward the top of the steps a group of people huddled. They were all wearing either traditional Bhutanese ghos or monk robes. Dorji jogged toward the group. I followed. As I quickly climbed the narrow stairs, I could see feet hanging from the edge of the steps.

A monk—shaved head, thin glasses, maroon robes—was down and unconscious. I recalled the basic emergency training I took and checked his spine for signs of fracture. Nothing. A general understanding arose within the group. The man needed to be moved to flat ground so he could be airlifted out.

The stairs were too steep and narrow for a group carry. So we carefully propped the monk onto the back of the largest person, who hoofed him down the steps. With the help of the group he laid the monk onto a flat grass patch along the cliffside trail.

The monk's eyes were rolled back, as if he were scrutinizing the brain above them. "I'm going to do CPR," I slowly told the group. They only partially understood me. As I knelt in front of him, two tiny women, a mother and a daughter who were both doctors in Hong Kong, were suddenly at my side. They'd been hiking to the monastery when they walked into this scene.

They pressed their fingers to the man's neck to check vitals and agreed that CPR was needed. These two were surely better trained. But I was the only person with any training who was also large enough to execute CPR optimally on the 200-pound monk.

I tore open his robe, revealing a gold T-shirt. I dug my knees into the dirt, overlapped my hands, and placed the heel of my right hand on the monk's sternum. Then I began hammering into his chest, 100 beats a minute, as the younger Hong Kong doctor started a timer.

I was unsure of the cultural implications of giving a monk mouth-to-mouth. So the daughter doctor quickly instructed one of the other monks, a woman, on how to do it. The woman monk breathed into him, repeatedly pushing air into his lungs. Then I was back to compressing his chest.

"Time is ten minutes, twenty-six seconds," said the daughter doctor. A crowd had formed around us, and a driver who was on the phone stepped into the group. "Helicopter cannot come," he told us. There was nowhere to land, and the cliffs were too close for an airlift.

The doctor checked the monk's vitals. She shook her head. I continued pressing. Pressing as hard as I could, thinking that if I could push hard enough it might kick-start his heart. We hit the 15-minute mark. His face was distant. "Twenty minutes, eleven seconds," said the doctor. "You can stop." He was gone.

Here was a man who just minutes ago had hiked five steep miles, joking and laughing and talking with friends along the way. Death can come at any time.

PART FIVE

Carry the load.

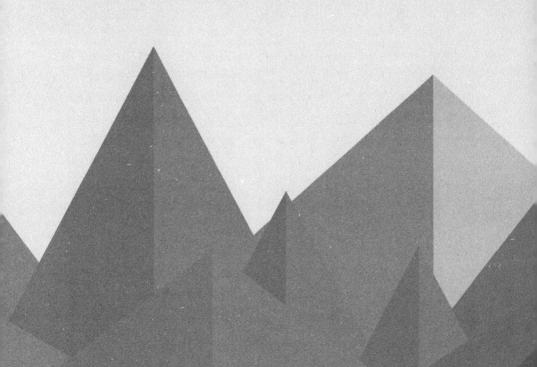

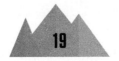

100+ POUNDS

THE MEAT IS dry, merlot-red, and resting in rows. There are two 50-pound hindquarters, two 35-pound front quarters, and about 70 pounds of backstraps, loins, neck meat, ribs, and more. The caribou's cape is laid out hair-side down on the tundra.

Donnie, William, and I stand surveying the spread. "The hunter should pack out the heaviest load," Donnie says. "And he always carries the head."

So it looks like I'll be getting the weighty end of the bargain. Donnie grabs a hindquarter, front quarter, and side of ribs and dumps them into his pack. William will take a front quarter, the rib section, and the backstraps, loins, and neck meat—a big ball of flesh.

I heave a hindquarter inside my pack. The cape's underside is smooth, white, and sticky like rubber as I roll it to fit into my pack. It's shockingly heavy for a bundle of hair, about 40 pounds, because of all of the water retained in the skin.

The caribou's head weighs about 20 pounds. It's placed neck down on the outside of my pack, as if the caribou is looking out behind me. I drop the bag's lid over the animal's forehead, and William steps over to help me crank down straps to secure the load.

Our packs all weigh between 90 and 110 pounds. Trying to muscle that weight up on our own is an efficient way to throw out a back or shoulder. So William and I as a team grab Donnie's pack, each holding open a strap so he can back in and secure the load tight on his shoulders.

Donnie and I do the same for William. Then it's my turn.

When the two release the load it rips me back a step. Subconscious, reactive impulses take over. I lock my entire body to save myself from falling butt-first onto the tundra.

Then I'm looking at what's left of the caribou: a fleshy spinal column, entrails, and hooves. Donnie asks, "Do you think you'd hunt again?"

"I don't know," I say.

He eyes me like he's expecting some kind of elaboration. But I have neither the desire nor the energy to get all contemplative. The weight of the pack is cutting into my shoulders and dragging on my hips, making even the basic act of breathing a struggle. And we haven't even started hiking the five miles back to camp.

As a sort of karmic penance for killing, the walk is entirely uphill. We'll face a mile or so of a slight pitch. It'll ramp upward into a grueling 20-degree hill for about a mile and a half. Then the land will lay off into a 10-degree slope for another mile and a half until we hit the ridge above camp, which we'll walk for one final mile.

So we start trudging, leaving the caribou's remains as a buffet for ravens, grizzlies, wolves, and, over time, lichen and moss.

Within 15 minutes Donnie is out front. William is ten yards behind him and I'm ten beyond that. The sun is sweeping across the horizon, casting my shadow long down the tundra. With the caribou's four-foot antlers bursting from my pack, my silhouette looks like some sort of mythical Arctic man-beast.

The weight is easier to manage with the pack's hip belt buckled tight. But only for a handful of minutes. My lower-body muscles eventually start feeling like they're being blowtorched off my bones. So I unbuckle the belt and let the blood rush down into my legs to relieve the acidy tension. This rides the weight entirely on my shoulders. Within a few minutes the shoulder straps feel like they're slowly cutting down my torso, slicing me lengthwise into thirds. So I switch back to the hip belt.

I'm also gripping the rifle at my side. Ten pounds isn't much. Until it is. Which is when my forearms feel ablaze. I switch hands often. All the while my lungs feel like they're sitting atop Bunsen burners.

These heavy back-and-forths continue, each transition successively more demanding.

The weight also amplifies the question of where to step. Tussock, mattress, muck, or shale? The 100-plus extra pounds can take one bad step and push it from a sprain into a fracture. Yet there is one upside of this mental puzzle. A study funded by the UK's Ministry of Defence discovered that people who engaged in a mentally demanding task while exercising increased their time to exhaustion a relative 300 percent more compared to a group who zoned out while doing the exact same 12-week exercise program.

We put one foot in front of the other at a pace of about a mile or two an hour. That's all we can physically muster. The combination of weight, undulating ground, and gradient unites into a blitzkrieg on the system.

Dense clouds are rolling in from the east.

"Looks like snow," yells William.

"The good news is, it's usually not as cold when it snows," shouts back Donnie.

The bad news: snow. Slippery, cold, wet snow.

Something occurs to me two hours into the trek, during the steepest section of hill. I've never worked this physically hard for this long. I've done efforts that were intense but quick. Like when I burned 60 calories in 60 seconds on a fan bike and afterward vomited. I've done efforts that were easier but far longer. Like a 24-hour unsupported endurance event. This act is a marriage between them. At once too intense and too long.

My heart rate is the same I'd have trying to run my fastest marathon. And the muscles in my legs and torso feel like they would during some really masochistic lower-body workout. Like German volume training—ten sets of ten heavy squats. Except that there is seemingly no upper limit on the reps and sets out here.

Perhaps even worse is that the whole endeavor is characterized by a looming, slightly terrifying catch. There is no way out. Unlike a marathon or a workout at the gym, I can't just decide I've had enough and veer off course into a 7-Eleven for a Snickers and a Slurpee, or choose to go easy on myself and grab lighter weights. I can hardly slow down, because I'm already walking at a zombie-like pace and the act is absolutely burying me. And the meat weighs what it weighs.

I stop occasionally. But removing the pack means I'll have to muscle the damn thing back up. The best way to "rest" is to place my hands on my thighs and bend forward so that my torso is parallel with the ground. The position shifts the weight's pressure for a moment, letting the lactic acid wash out. Then it's back to walking.

We walk in silence. Not because we don't want to talk. But rather because we're all breathing too heavily, all burrowed too deeply in our own respective pain caves and trying to silence our brains, which are screaming at us to stop, slow down, take a seat, quit.

Well, mine is, anyway. William seems slightly better off than me. Donnie, up in front, is confidently striding with his eyes up and taking in the view. The guy wouldn't impress anyone in a serious gym. But put him out here and he's an elite human pack mule.

I think about what Marcus Elliott said about exploring the boundaries of our comfort zones. "In misogi you'll reach this edge where you are convinced you have nothing left," he said. "But you'll keep going anyway. And then you'll look back and you'll be way out beyond what you were certain was your edge. You won't forget that." The human brain may hate failure, but it hates exercise equally so.

Humans over millennia developed a complex network of physical discomforts and psychological "governors" to dissuade us from effort, because effort requires energy, or calories, which in the past was precious. This is why we seemingly have an ingrained call to laziness.

When a person does physical labor their muscles demand more oxygen, which their body must work to deliver. This causes a faster heart rate and heavier breaths, leading to burning sensations in our lungs. When we lift and carry things, the energy-burning by-product lactate builds up in our muscles. This makes them gradually feel like they're engulfed in flames. If an early human had felt orgasmic pleasure through, say, carrying heavy rocks uphill, she would have quickly burned through all her energy stores and died.

Exercise physiologists up until the end of the 21st century believed that physical exhaustion was simply a matter of supply and demand. But the theory didn't seem to match reality. No one had ever proved that muscles were getting too little oxygen or fuel. What's more, studies showed that when people hit the wall during prolonged exercise, they were recruiting only a fraction of their muscle fibers.

Sometime in the mid 1990s, a new idea eventually occurred to Timothy Noakes, MD, PhD, director of the Exercise Science and Sports Medicine Research Unit at the University of Cape Town. He thought that because we activate muscle by way of our brain, our brain must also be responsible for determining how long, hard, and fast we push ourselves. He called the idea the "central governor theory," and began conducting research. Over three decades he's shown that exercise-induced fatigue is predominantly a protective *emotion*. It's a psychological state that has little to do with a person's physical limits.

One study on the theory analyzed the fMRI brain activity of cyclists as they pedaled to exhaustion. "We saw that the limbic lobe— the emotional center of the brain—lit up as the intensity increased and the cyclists became more exhausted," Edward Fontes, PhD, the lead researcher told me. "The more active the limbic lobe became, the more emotion they tied to exertion and the more they slowed."

The brain uses the "unpleasant [but illusory] sensations of fatigue" to pump the body's brakes well before a person comes close to real physical exhaustion, Noakes discovered. Which explains Elliott's observations on limits.

To take my mind off the discomfort, I settle into a respiratory rhythm. I take one step as I breathe in, then two steps as I breathe out. One step breathing in, two steps breathing out. Over and over, focusing only on the breath.

There's science behind this. Brazilian researchers found that people who are able to detach from their emotions during exercise—for example, not thinking about or putting a negative valence on their burning lungs and legs—almost always perform better. And I'll take whatever I can get right now.

At some point, shale appears beneath my feet and we've reached the top of a mesa. Its lesser incline is a relative relief. I pause and stand tall, sucking down a cold breath of Arctic air.

I'VE EXERCISED ABOUT FIVE HOURS A WEEK FOR NEARLY TWO DECADES. BUT I'VE never put my body through anything like this expedition. The trip exposed a flaw not only in my own physicality but also in how the modern world approaches fitness. Compared to humans of the recent past, I'd be the last person picked in gym class.

Before we figured out animal husbandry and crop cultivation we were "essentially professional athletes whose livelihood required [us] to be physically active," said Harvard anthropologists. Our ancestors didn't "work out," because nearly all of their waking hours were spent doing things that today we would classify as exercise.

Early humans walked and ran long distances across untamed earth. Studies show it was not uncommon for these hunters to run and walk more than 25 miles in a day. We call that a marathon. They called it "picking up dinner."

They were usually carrying items as they covered this rough ground. Mostly stuff that weighed between 5 and 20 pounds, like tools, weapons, water jugs, food, babies, etc. But sometimes the loads were like what I'm lugging in Alaska. For example, a hindquarter of a zebra—an animal today still pursued by African hunter-gatherers—typically weighs about 80 pounds. And the hunters didn't pack it out with some ergonomic backpack. They slung the limb over a shoulder, Fred Flintstone–style, and hoofed it home.

To find foods like tubers, early humans had to dig a few feet into the ground. This act would take at least 30 minutes of strenuous work and could burn anywhere from 200 to 300 calories. They climbed trees and cliffs for honey. They threw projectiles fast and hard. They fought enemies and beasts to the death.

Even doing nothing wasn't effortless. Our ancestors often rested in the squat position, which required they lightly activate nearly every muscle in their body or else topple over. Or they sat or slept on the ground, which, given its rough nature, forced them to shift around frequently as positions became too uncomfortable. This constant shifting and fidgeting to find comfort while at rest can burn as many as 400 more calories across a day compared to sitting stationary, according to research from the Mayo Clinic.

David Raichlen is an anthropologist at the University of Southern California. Picture a darker and more chiseled version of Matt Damon. Like Damon when he's in shape to play Jason Bourne. Raichlen has spent a lot of time in the African bush studying Hadza hunter-gatherers to understand the exercise of our forefathers and how it impacted their health and physiology.

"We've used different ways of measuring their physical activity," he said. "We've used accelerometers [step counters] on their thighs and wrists, we've used heart rate data, we've used GPS."

Raichlen, along with colleagues in a series of studies, had tribe members wear GPS activity-tracking watches and tested their metabolisms. He wanted to know how much the people move and how many calories they burn a day. He also gathered the same information from everyday Americans.

The team quickly observed one obvious difference between these two groups: the Americans were much larger. The men in the tribe weigh an average of 112 pounds and the women weigh 95. The American men and women, meanwhile, clocked in at 179 and 164 pounds.

The satellite data showed that the Hadza men covered about 9 daily miles. Sometimes, like during a hunt, that number could jump well past 20 miles. All their physical work—walking, carrying, digging, climbing—caused the men to burn an average of 2,649 calories a day.

The calorie burn of the American men, meanwhile, averaged 3,053. And so it may appear that the Americans had an edge. The numbers, however, are all relative.

The data showed that the Hadza men every day burned about 24 calories per pound of their body weight. The American men, with their far more sedentary lives, burned just 17. The same finding was shown for the women. Hadza women burned 20 calories per pound of their body weight, while American women burned about 14. Pound for pound, the Hadza burn more than 40 percent more calories a day than Westerners.

The US government recommends that Americans each week get 150 minutes of what they call "moderate to vigorous physical activity," or MVPA. Less than half of Americans manage this 20 or so minutes a day of exercise. And, like, vacuuming and mowing the lawn count as MVPA.

"But if you look at total MVPA of the Hadza, they're [getting] well over two hundred minutes *a day*," said Raichlen. Other people who live like our ancestors are equally active. The Tsimane tribe in the Bolivian rain forest and the Ache in Paraguay, for example, each walk more than ten daily miles. And they're also doing the same other endurance and strength-heavy, necessary-in-order-not-to-die physical tasks.

Only 20 percent of Americans meet the national guidelines for weekly endurance and strength exercise. And 27 percent of us don't do any type of physical activity at all. Literally nothing—life as a sort of prolonged shuffle from bed to office chair to sofa to bed.

This, along with our jones for ultraprocessed foods, is why research from the CDC shows that we modern humans are fatter and less muscular than we were a decade ago. Which was when we were fatter and less muscular than we were the decade before that, and so on. Scientists say our impossible laziness—once exceedingly rare—is leading to dangerously low levels of muscle. This condition is called sarcopenia, which is the loss of muscle mass and function, and it's now creeping into younger populations for the first time in any species in all of history. Humans are slowly becoming as unique for our fatness and lack of fitness as we are for our intelligence.

The numbers suggest that our forefathers in just three-quarters of a day logged more activity than most of us now do in a week or two. And they basically stayed at this activity level until they died.

"In hunter-gatherer tribes even the older adults are getting unbelievably high levels of physical activity," said Raichlen. One of his colleagues wrote that "80-year-old grandmothers are still strong and vital."

"They have no other option [but to stay active], really," said Raichlen. If a person couldn't sustain activity and contribute to resource allocation, they simply wouldn't survive. Today being radically out of shape, no matter a person's age, rarely results in a quick death. But it often does result in chronic conditions like heart disease and diabetes that cause a slow death.

Even modern athletes are unimpressive compared to a run-of-the-mill ancient. The arms of the average prehistoric woman, for example, were 16 percent stronger than those of today's Olympic rowers, according to scientists at the University of Cambridge. Other research shows that the average prehistoric Joe had an "ability to just keep going" equal to the endurance of today's elite college cross-country athletes. And prehistoric Joe didn't have Nike sponsorships,

performance meal plans, supplements, and scientific training programs. He did, however, have hunger.

This is why some authors and thinkers have argued that ancient
and modern hunter-gatherers are like some sort of superhuman athletic freaks. But that's just not true, according to scientists at Harvard. The researchers call this problematic viewpoint "the fallacy of
the athletic savage." Our ancestors and modern tribes were and are
just like every other *Homo sapien.* The truth is, every human body
can achieve amazing physical feats when it's forced to.

How'd we become the least fit humans of all time? "Technologies
often end up reducing our physical activity levels," said Raichlen.
This truth extends even to the Hadza. They provide the best activity model for the earliest humans, but they're likely *less* active than
hunter-gatherers of the past.

"The Hadza use projectile weapons for hunting. The earliest African hunter-gatherers didn't have projectile weapons," said Raichlen.
Instead of shooting an arrow from a distance, early humans likely
carried out persistence hunts, running down their kill to the point of
exhaustion over miles and miles.

Kalahari bushmen in fact used the technique as recently as a decade ago, until South Africa banned hunting altogether, according to
Louis Liebenberg, an evolutionary biologist at Harvard. Liebenberg
discovered that Kalahari persistence hunts required the bushmen to
run an average 9:40 minutes per mile pace across more than 20 miles
of rugged, sandy terrain in 107 degrees Fahrenheit.

The first great change in human physicality began with the advent of farming about 13,000 years ago. Studies show that prehistoric farmers, for example, were fitter than their ancestors in some
ways but not others. They had stronger upper bodies from grinding grain and tilling soil but relatively weak lower bodies because
they covered long distances in search of food less often. But the
data shows that early farmers were at least as active as early hunter-
gatherers. Most of humanity rather quickly transitioned to farming,

and at least 80 percent of civilized people were farmers until the next big shift.

The second great change in human fitness began around 1850. It marked the start of the Industrial Revolution, and today just 13.7 percent of jobs require the same heavy work as our past days of farming. Roughly three-quarters of jobs are now sedentary, and we're sitting more every year. Over the last decade, the average American added another hour of daily sitting. Adults now sit for six and a half hours, while kids sit more than eight (the removal of recess hasn't helped, either). And we don't sit like our ancestors, squatting and being forced to move around. We melt into plush chairs that require no muscle activation.

When we fully transitioned to effortless work, we did so with those hardwired patterns that favor laziness and make us far less likely to recoup our lost movement. A figure that shows just how predisposed humans are to default to comfort: 2. That's the percent of people who take the stairs when they also have the option to take an escalator.

As the effects of our inactivity began mounting—JFK called us "soft Americans" in 1960—we made an attempt to add lost movement back into our days. But we did a rather shitty job on the engineering end.

Forget ridiculous vibrating belts, sweatsuits, and *8-Minute Abs* tapes. Health clubs became a staple of society beginning in the 1960s and '70s. These gave us cardio and weight machines, Zumba classes, etc. Exercise was no longer a fact of life. It became a 30-minute class or hourlong session we tackled a few times a week. A separate and distinct time to try to recoup lost movement.

Exercise is never exactly comfortable, but the average gym attempts to make it so. A typical workout for most people today is zoning out to reality TV while running along a motorized belt in a temperature-controlled room. Another popular machine has users make repetitive elliptical motions with their arms and legs—motions never occurring until the advent of that machine.

Or we sit on a padded seat, resting our joints against another pad, and move ergonomic handles attached to a stack of weights along a fixed movement path. Another situation that is physically easier than anything we'd ever face in nature, and that neglects important stabilizing muscles.

In the free-weight room we lift perfectly balanced weights of our choosing a predetermined number of times. But research shows that the awkwardly shaped objects our ancestors lifted worked far more muscles compared to the balanced weights we lift at the gym. And we lifted those loads until the job was done.

Many people in fact strive to build gargantuan levels of muscle just for the sake of it. Piling on muscle throughout the timeline of our species would have been not only impossible, thanks to resource allocation, but also a dangerous liability—hunting and evading predators required fantastic speed and endurance. Our lifestyles made us strong but didn't bulk us up. This is why average-size people who are exceedingly strong are said to possess "farm-boy strength." "Gym strength," on the other hand, is a criticism of people who look fit but suffer under real physical labor.

When we took our workouts indoors, we also lost a critical brain stimulus, according to research conducted by Raichlen and published in *Trends in Neuroscience.*

"Hunting and foraging is not just a physical exercise, it's a cognitive one," said Raichlen. As we walked, ran, carried, dug, or climbed, we were also taxing our brain's motor control, memory, spatial navigation, and executive functioning, he said. He describes past humans as "cognitively engaged 'endurance athletes.'" Over time the exercise of mind and body created a symbiotic relationship, where the combination of physical and mental work improved neural responses and brain health.

When I spoke with Liebenberg I asked him what people most often get wrong about hunter-gatherers. I expected him to say diet, because the popular paleo diet is regularly criticized by PhD-wielding anthropologists. But he surprised me. "Everyone thinks persistence hunting is purely a physical act," he said. "We underestimate the intellectual side of it." As the bushmen run, they must also consider animal behavior and biology, land patterns, tracking, pacing, and far more.

"A lot of exercise we do now is indoors, in a gym," said Raichlen. "There's a lot of work to be done to see just how cognitively challenging it is to sit on an exercise bike for half an hour."

Any and all activity, indoor or otherwise, is great. "[Gym cardio] is certainly stressing your cardiovascular system, and that has brain benefits. But is it reflective of how our physiology is best adapted to exercise?" said Raichlen. "If you put people outside, like if you're going for a bike ride or trail run, where you're having to navigate, make decisions about when to stop, how to pace, where to turn . . . all of those things add a cognitive challenge to that activity." And that, Raichlen believes, could enhance and protect the human brain—sharpening it, making it quicker and more disease resistant.

In the paper Raichlen wrote, "When faced with chronic inactivity over the lifespan, as is common in modern industrialized societies . . . [our] lack of either exercise in general or cognitive demands during exercise may lead to capacity reductions or suboptimal capacity maintenance in the brain similar to those seen in other organ systems. . . . Our brains adaptively reduce capacity as part of an energy-saving strategy, leading to age-related brain atrophy."

When we do exercise outside, it's often spent running in cushioned shoes along a perfectly paved road. This act burns more calories than running on the equivalent gym machine. But not as many as running on raw earth. Biomechanists at the University of Michigan discovered that the increased challenge of walking or running on untamed, uneven ground forces people to burn an average of 28 percent more energy per step compared to paved ground.

Whenever we feel tired or bored we sit and rest. Or take a cool drink of filtered water. Or change the song on our smartphone.

When our predetermined time, distance, or set and rep scheme is up, we can go sit in a sauna.

The answer isn't going back to days spent working for our food rather than for a paycheck. Our comfortable world is great. But our tip into comfort has created a world that rarely presents us with physical challenges, and we have, in turn, paid for it with our health and hardiness.

PACKING OUT THE CARIBOU FEELS ODDLY PRIMEVAL. IT'S A UNIQUE MARRIAGE OF strength and endurance that is foreign coming from the modern fitness world. Humans today rarely do one of the most consequential acts of our forefathers: carrying heavy stuff over rough land. But emerging research is showing that it's an act that made us human.

"We're getting there, boys," says William.

From atop the mesa we can see miles in every direction. The storm is closing in from the east. The Brooks Range mountains are psychedelic white pyramids in the northeast. A raven floats overhead. Donnie stops 20 yards up front, and William and I close the gap.

He points southwest, where the mesa curves and rises into a butte. At its base are two Dall sheep, a young ewe and ram. Both are frozen and staring directly at us. The male's horns are perhaps a foot long and just beginning to curve. Lean muscle striations under his white coat pop in the light. "Those two have probably never seen humans before," says Donnie.

"Well, to be honest, I've never seen a Dall sheep before," I say.

Our two groups stare at each other for another minute. Then the dull aching in my shoulders and legs brings me back to the task at hand.

We have another mile to go. Just 5,280 more feet.

20

≤50 POUNDS

OUR ANCESTORS STARTED walking on two feet, like we do, about 4.4 million years ago. There are about a dozen theories why. But researchers are in agreement that the evolutionary advantages accruing from the ability to carry objects—food or otherwise—played a principal role.

Four-legged animals can't carry well. (Unless, like pack animals, a human straps the weight onto them.) They have to carry or drag items with their mouth, which they can't do for any appreciable distance.

Primates are unique because we can carry stuff in our hands while we cover ground with our feet. Monkeys, apes, etc., generally suck at this, though. They tend to carry short distances, because for them the act is highly inefficient. It costs a chimp 75 percent more energy to walk the same distance as a human. Which is why those animals mostly cover ground on four limbs and "knuckle walk," as anthropologists call it.

When monkeys walk upright it's with a tipsy, bent-knee, bent-hip gait. Their upper body sways from side to side with each step. Add weight to that wonky walk and it becomes even more inefficient. Humans, on the other hand, can carry up to 15 percent of our body weight—roughly 30 pounds for an average male—and we still use less energy than other primates, even when they're not carrying anything.

Chimps also struggle to grasp and side-carry loads that are just a few pounds. But humans can easily grip heavy weights and walk. Research shows that it's difficult but totally doable for an average male to side-carry 75 pounds.

After visiting with Rachel Hopman in Boston, I strolled up to Harvard. I met with Dan Lieberman, one of the world's leading anthropologists and a professor at the university. Lieberman studies the evolution of the human body and why we're built the way we are, especially as it relates to movement and physicality.

His office was Ivy League bordering on cliché. Expansive with lots of oak, way too many academic crests, overstuffed bookshelves, and rich leather couches and chairs that surrounded a coffee table lined with scientific journals. It was at the top floor of Harvard's Peabody Museum of Archaeology and Ethnology (think: a place where Indiana Jones might store his finds).

Anthropologists since the discipline's inception had always believed running played a minimal role in how humans evolved. They considered it something of a useless parlor trick.

The notion made sense. It costs humans twice as much energy to sprint compared to other mammals, and our two legs and upright posture make us pretty slow. The fastest a human has ever covered 100 meters, for example, is in 9.58 seconds. That required an average speed of about 23 miles an hour. And the runner could only sustain that for another handful of meters.

For comparison, a pronghorn antelope can hit 55 miles an hour. A grizzly can do 35. Even the poodle Paris Hilton keeps in her purse can run 30. And those animals can run at those speeds for minutes at a time. We're also terrible jumpers, jukers, lifters, and climbers. We two-legged mammals are indeed, as Lieberman puts it, "athletically pathetic."

But in 2004 he released a study that shook the foundations of both the anthropology and exercise communities. Lieberman found that, no, we can't go fast. But we can go far—especially in hot weather. The freaks among us can sustain speeds as high as 13 miles an hour for distances over 25 miles. Think: professional marathoners. But even hobbyist runners every weekend finish marathons in three to four hours, averaging about 9 to 6.5 miles an hour. On a hot day a relatively fit human will beat every other mammal in a distance race—lions, tigers, bears, dogs, etc.*

As Lieberman explained in his *Nature* paper, nicknamed "Born to Run,"† humans can do this thanks to a handful of adaptations we developed over millions of years. We stand on two legs and have springy arches in our feet, long tendons in our legs, big butt muscles, sweat glands across our body, no fur, complicated noses that humidify air before it hits our lungs—the list goes on. These help us run great distances and stay cool while doing it. Other mammals gallop quickly for a few minutes, then need to stop and pant to release heat and cool down.

Endurance was our killer app and as we evolved we used it to our advantage on hot days with persistence hunting: slowly but surely tracking and running down prey for miles upon miles until the animal toppled over from heat exhaustion. Then we'd spear or club it and have dinner.

Lieberman's paper also suggested that human running mechanics fundamentally changed with the introduction of cushiony, comfortable running shoes in the 1970s. Those shoes typically lead a person to first strike the ground with their heel. Early humans running barefoot likely first struck the ground with the middle or front of their feet. This original foot-striking pattern, according to Lieberman and other anthropologists' work, may be more efficient and reduce common running injuries. Lieberman is the man who planted the seed from which the "barefoot running" movement grew. (Although he's

---

* This rule does not hold in cold weather. In cold weather, sled dogs are by far the best endurance athletes. They can run 100 miles a day for days on end, running sub-four-minute miles most of the time. Caribou aren't bad, either. Put either of those animals near the Equator, though, and they're toast.

† A decade later, journalist Chris McDougall would borrow the line for the title of his bestselling book about barefoot running.

quick to point out that he's not a barefoot-running "advocate," just a guy who studies it.)

I was familiar with Lieberman's running work. But while training to hoof heavy weight across Alaska, I had contacted him to ask if he knew of any research on early humans' capacity for load carrying. He was, in fact, investigating that exact topic in his lab and invited me to meet with him. So there I was in his office following up on strength and what role it played for early humans.

"Strength is interesting," Lieberman said. "Because there's a lot of ideas out there about how important strength is. I think it's often driven by what people like. There are a lot of people out there who love being in the gym and lifting weights and dislike aerobic activity. They often pump up just how good resistance training is relative to aerobic training. And the reverse is also true. People who do aerobic training and don't like being in the gym are often dismissive of the importance of strength, right? It's kind of a Rorschach test. Obviously strength and endurance are both important." We perform and advocate for the exercise we're most comfortable with.

"But . . ." He paused. "I think the balance of evidence is that humans have undergone intense selection for endurance and aerobic activity and that strength is not as important in humans as it is in some other species." Male chimpanzees, for example, are far smaller yet twice as strong as even the most buff humans. Athletically pathetic, indeed.

"It seems [our ancestors] had just enough strength for day-to-day tasks," said Lieberman. "There's published data that suggest that hunter-gatherers are moderately strong. But they're not like today's gym rats in any sense. Like, where would they find a bench press?"

Our most radical strength feats were muscling loads great distances over rough ground. Humans are, in fact, "extreme" in their ability to move items from point A to B, wrote researchers in a study in the journal *PLOS One*.

And natural selection over time seems to have picked humans who were the best, most efficient carriers, found a study in the *Journal of Anatomy*. Carrying, the research suggests, is a driving force behind why we became apex predators.

The more we ran down prey, carried it long distances back home, then feasted, the more we were shaped into who we are today. The majority of the adaptations that help us run far in the heat also helped us carry far. Our legs, for example, became comparatively longer while our torsos became shorter and stronger, better to locomote while loaded down. And the reason we can "lock" our hand bones into our wrist bones and generate abnormally strong forces with our middle finger is so we can grab heavy stuff and hoof it.

Early humans may not have been great at bench presses. But the animal weights they carried could be radically heavy. A review in *Evolutionary Anthropology* found that the animals we hunted ranged in size from 22 to 5,500 pounds. The average weighed about 220 to 770 pounds. Which means that the butchered hindquarters, front quarters, backstraps, loins, neck meat, and ribs were not exactly light loads. Particularly since we hauled them for miles without packs.

Archaeological evidence also shows that humans were transporting heavy rocks to make tools with as early as 2.6 million years ago. One site in Israel revealed that our ancestors carried 90-pound stones short distances. But other sites show they hauled lighter boulders nearly ten miles. Early humans had "a willingness to carry stone for hours," wrote the scientists.

These people carried their belongings when they moved camp, too. (Perhaps to camp at the body of that 5,500-pound animal.) An analysis of 36 different hunter-gatherer tribes showed that many moved camp a few hundred miles each year. The Innu tribe of northeast Canada essentially lived as professional movers. They covered an average of 2,200 miles a year over their frequent moves.

Carrying, as I was learning in Alaska, is uncomfortable. It's an act that kills the division between strength and cardio. It jams a person into an exhausting feedback loop. The walking makes the weight feel heavier. The weight makes the walking more of a lung buster.

But it shaped us. And, in fact, carrying was likely more common than running. Running was reserved mostly for hunts. But to gather we'd amble away from camp and then carry back what we found. Most of these loads were small, likely 10 to 20 pounds. But scientists in Spain say gatherers sometimes carry weights equal to half of their total body weight.

So it seems that humans were perhaps even more so "born to carry." And like its brother running, our need to carry was largely rendered moot by tech. We have shopping carts, wheeled suitcases, strollers, vehicles, dollies, semitrucks, forklifts, etc.

Unlike running, most of us never reengineered carrying back into our days. There is, however, one modern tribe that hasn't forgotten it. They've embraced it. Their lives, in fact, depend on their ability to move loads. And it's helped them become perhaps the fittest band of humans ever to walk the earth.

IT WAS 7:45 ON A BALMY WINTER MORNING IN ATLANTIC BEACH, FLORIDA, AND I WAS standing in Jason McCarthy's front yard.

His bright white two-story, aqua-shuttered house is a block from the Atlantic Ocean. Salty air was winding up the tucked-away street as McCarthy bent down, picked up his three-year-old son, Ryan, and strapped him into a stroller. McCarthy then slung on a sparely designed black CORDURA backpack filled with his laptop, a PB&J, and a 45-pound steel plate. The weight was weight for the sake of it. Heavy to be heavy.

He then grabbed an identical-weight plate and slid it inside an identical black pack. "There's yours," he said. "Let's go."

I muscled it over my back and had to flex my legs and stomach to resist the weight's awkward pull. Then we began walking the palm-lined street. Our pace felt decently comfortable despite the heavy pack. Until McCarthy looked at his wristwatch. "Oh," he said. "We need to hurry a bit. I have a meeting at nine." Our mission: travel five miles to HQ by way of Ryan's preschool.

McCarthy extended his arms to create distance between his body and the stroller, then began something faster than a walk but slower than a run, one foot always maintaining ground contact. "We call this a ruck shuffle," he said. Picture a slightly hunched combo of jogging and fast walking.

"Ruck" is both a noun and a verb. It's a thing and an action. It's military-speak for the heavy backpack that carries all of the items a soldier needs to fight a war. And "to ruck" or "rucking" is the act of marching that ruck in war, or as a form of training for soldiers or civilians to get really, really fit.

"You very rarely run in war, and never without weight. Never," said McCarthy. "But you're *always* rucking."

McCarthy's legs unfurled one after the other. The movement accentuated his build: six foot four and 190 pounds. All length. No fat. With a layer of lean muscle coating him from head to toe. Picture Disney's Ichabod Crane if Ichabod Crane were a Green Beret. Which McCarthy happens to be.

He served from 2003 to 2008, during which time he was deployed to Iraq and Africa. The army wasn't the original plan.

After graduating from college, McCarthy dreamed of doing James Bond–type stuff for the CIA. But a year into the recruiting process an agent had bad news. "We don't train agents for special operations," the agent said. "We just recruit those guys from military Special Forces units, where they've already been trained."

Thanks for the year-late heads-up, McCarthy said, then enlisted with the hopes of making it into the Special Forces. "When I first got to the military I didn't know what rucking was. In infantry school they handed me a heavy ruck and the advice was basically 'keep up,'" said McCarthy. Next was Airborne School. Then Special Forces preparation, assessment, and selection. That took him to the qualification course, a 53-week curriculum of learning and suffering.

"Getting yelled at while doing group workouts is what people see in documentaries about Special Forces Selection and Assessment. But that's, like, four hours of three weeks. It's actually much quieter than that," he said. "The missions would be, 'Here's a map, a compass, and your ruck. Get to this destination.' The ruck had to be forty-five pounds dry. The rule was 'Don't be late, light, or last.'"

McCarthy would need to quickly cover anywhere from 10 to 20 miles through the North Carolina pine forests alone in the dark with only his thoughts and ruck. "So I'd move in a ruck shuffle. Faster than what we're doing now," he said.

And what we were doing had in just ten minutes caused sweat to percolate down our faces and drip off our chins. McCarthy and I weren't lollygagging, but it seemed like we were still going to be late. So he pushed the pace.

"Left," he said, steering the stroller onto Ocean Street, a beach-bum street filled with seafood restaurants and nautical-themed bars.

At the end of his training came Robin Sage, the litmus test for those hoping to earn the Green Beret. Soldiers are placed in small teams and air-dropped into the middle of the woods at night for the ultimate test of their ability to conduct unconventional warfare. The military creates a statewide, live-action exercise in guerrilla war, where other soldiers play the enemy and fire blank rounds. "Everyone's ruck weighed a hundred and twenty-five pounds, plus we had equipment," he said. "Then we had to do an eighteen-hour infiltration. You can't think. You can barely move."

McCarthy said, "I began to feel like the ruck was an extension of my body. My bones were denser. I was leaner and stronger. My endurance was through the roof." The army shipped the newly minted Green Beret to Iraq and the ruck never left.

Anthropologists like Lieberman are understanding that carrying was likely fundamental to human evolution. But historians have long known that humans carry during vitally human acts, like hunting, exploring, and fighting.

We know that the earliest hunters carried items like spears, clubs, and hopefully meat. Exploratory expeditions, beginning with the Phoenicians in 1550 BC, carried survival resources into the unknown. If successful, they'd haul back precious spices, metals, information, and more.

"And in the military you're always carrying weight. No matter what. Always," said McCarthy. "Rucking is the foundational skill of being a Special Forces soldier. Any soldier for that matter."

Prehistoric cave art depicts warriors heading into tribal battles with crude shields and spears. Together these items could weigh 10 to 20 pounds. Thousands of years ago Greek hoplites, Roman legionaries, and Byzantine infantrymen all marched with around 30 pounds of gear. Fighters in all regiments around the world until the mid-1800s, in fact, carried between 20 and 35 pounds.

Then British soldiers in the Crimean War began carrying an average of 65 pounds. Loads crept successively higher in World Wars I and II, Korea, and Vietnam. By the time America was engaged in Iraq and Afghanistan, the typical soldier was marching with about 100 pounds.

In the aftermath of the Crimean War, British scientists investigated the impacts of a soldier's load on his ability to fight war. Any infantryman, they found, could move quickly and safely marching with 50 pounds. About 150 years later, in the 2000s, three different studies from the US Army, Marines, and Navy all confirmed the finding. Fifty pounds is the heaviest load that allows soldiers to fight like hell, become physically bulletproof, and forge elite strength and endurance. This is why the military and industry are now looking for ways to lighten a soldier's load and rethinking training sessions that involve 100-pound rucks.

"Through time you've always had a warrior class that is at the physical tip of the spear," said McCarthy. "The Greeks, Roman legions, etc., they all trained similarly: load a rucksack and head out into the woods. US Special Forces trains this way. And the distance physically between the warrior class and the average citizen used to be small. But now that gap is wider than ever in human history.

"At the tip of the spear in the US we have the fittest soldiers who ever existed. At the opposite end we have the most unfit citizenry," he said. "And that is to our detriment and to the detriment of America."

Rucking is essential to military might. So the US government has poured millions of dollars into studying the act. McCarthy has read all this research and become something of a rucking-obsessed lay scientist. He's traveled the country to speak to physiologists, doctors, and government representatives to understand what rucking does to the human body.

"Rucking is strength and cardio in one," McCarthy said. "It's cardio for the person who hates running, and strength work for the person who hates lifting."

"So then what kind of body type does it build?" I asked.

"We call it super medium," he said. "Just think of Special Forces guys. We can't be too thin, but we also can't be too muscular. Rucking corrects for body type. Have too much fat or muscle? It'll lean you out. Too skinny? You'll get stronger and put on some muscle." This claim was recently confirmed in a study conducted by a team of researchers in Sweden. And data from the US Special Operations Command shows that the average operator weighs 175 solid pounds.

A casual ruck burns somewhere between two and three times the calories of walking, according to scientists at the University of South Carolina.

"But based on how voracious I am after a long, heavy ruck, I think it burns more than what many of the studies say," McCarthy said. "After long rucks in training I would sit down with a jar of peanut butter and eat a third of it. Then I'd pour M&Ms and granola in the jar, mix it, and finish the entire thing. I'd still lose weight."

A more accurate number may lie in declassified data presented at a summit on military physiology. It shows that the caloric burn of rucking unsurprisingly rises or falls based on a variety of factors: speed, load, and the type and slope of the terrain. The estimates suggest that what McCarthy did in Green Beret training in the North Carolina woods burned between 1,500 and 2,250 calories an hour. It also suggests that packing 100 pounds of caribou across the steepest pitches of the tundra burns between 1,850 and 2,150 an hour.

Rucking taxes the body's tactical chassis. That's according to Rob Shaul, who owns the Mountain Tactical Institute, a research and training center that develops fitness plans for mountain athletes and military operators. The tactical chassis is everything between the shoulders and knees: hamstrings, quads, hips, abs, obliques, back, etc. And rucking works this chassis as an integrated system. A strong, resilient tactical chassis is critical for overall fitness and injury resistance, particularly in hunting, and all combat and mountain sports.

"Hi, Janine!" McCarthy yelled as we approached an intersection.

"Hi, Jason!" yelled a middle-aged crossing guard, raising a stop sign as she barged into oncoming traffic.

We continued the ruck shuffle across the highway past a lineup of halted commuter traffic. The drivers looked somewhere between amused and worried that we were a guerrilla army invading the town. We arrived at Ryan's Montessori school after shuffling another tenth of a mile. McCarthy confiscated Ryan's preschool contraband—a bag of peanut-filled trail mix he'd been snacking on—then handed him off.

After 15 more minutes with boots on the ground, McCarthy and I reached our destination: GORUCK HQ.

The company resides in The George R. Lucier Jr. Building, a 1968 brick structure that sits two blocks from the ocean. I entered the main office, an expansive, brick-walled room. The walls were dotted with framed military photographs and movie posters. A six- by ten-foot American flag hung on a back wall.

There were four clusters of desks. Behind each computer sat either a seemingly everyday desk worker or a heavily tattooed ex–Special Forces soldier. All were fit and super medium.

McCarthy founded GORUCK after exiting the military. "Special Forces guys get all the best gear," he told me, pulling off his ruck. "You usually can't ruck with over thirty-five pounds in a regular backpack. I wanted to create a ruck that was to military specs but would look good in New York City. Something you could take to the office then toss some weight in and go for a ruck after work."

So he did. Took him about three years to develop the first GORUCK bag. It was a black, made-in-America, 26-liter ruck that could hold more weight than a person could ever carry in it.

His first customers were military guys, who'd use the rucks on raids in Kirkuk and Fallujah. Word spread and requests from America's elite soldiers steadily poured in. But McCarthy had a harder time reaching the average American. "I thought the world would just line up to buy my rucks," he said. "But they don't teach rucking in PE."

So he developed this far-out idea to get the word out about his company. His business smarts were novice, he said, "but I knew how to do military stuff."

He called it the GORUCK Challenge. With no less than 35 pounds in their rucks, people would as a team ruck for 12 hours across 15 to 20 miles. Along the way they'd complete group challenges assigned to them by McCarthy. Those challenges might entail team carrying of a 300-pound log for a mile or doing a ruck workout in the surf on a beach. A quarter-million people have now gone through GORUCK events. They've each been led by one of 250 combat-decorated Special Forces soldiers: SEALs, Green Berets, Rangers, Delta Force, MARSOC, etc.

There are also hundreds of "ruck clubs" across the world. These rucking converts have lost thousands of pounds, become physically stronger, and built active communities. They've also done some edge surfing, as Elliott called it—GORUCK offers events ranging from 6 to 48 hours.

"I've found that challenge and doing hard things is actually part of American DNA. It's like Kennedy said, 'We choose to go to the moon . . . and do the other things not because they are easy, but because they are hard,'" said McCarthy. "But we've now become a victim of the success of our species. There's been a rejection of physically hard things these days. Mostly because everything has become so easy that any difficulty is a bridge too far.

"Ask any SF guy: Doing physically hard things is an enormous life hack. Do hard things and the rest of life gets easier and you appreciate it all the more," McCarthy said. "Not doing physically hard things gets us all out of whack. The data is overwhelming in terms of our need to sweat, to be outside, to be part of a community. I'm not saying anything new here. I'm just reminding us of how we're hardwired. What's new today is that physically hard stuff is a novelty. Right, Mocha?"

"Damn straight" was the reply from a tattooed, weathered late-40-something at one of the desks. He's called Mocha for his daily eight-espresso-shot mochaccino habit. I'd later learn that another of his nicknames is The Million Dollar Man, for the grand total of all the hardware the US government had to install in his body after his 30-year career running special ops.

This idea was echoed to me recently by one of my best friends, William Allen, a former major in the US Marines and co-founder of Harpoon Ventures, a fast-rising defense-focused venture capital firm. "If you can consciously put yourself through physical discomfort and understand the higher purpose of it, the 'why,' the mental calluses that come along with that create what is called the Well of Fortitude," he said. "My business partner, who happens to be a prior service US Navy SEAL, and I were able to successfully build a legitimate venture capital fund from the ground up. Not because we were special, supersmart, or had access to family money. But rather, we knew our higher purpose and were able to draw on the Well of Fortitude we built on challenging missions in the military to buffer stress, work harder, and simply endure."

———

IT'S NOT JUST ELITE SOLDIERS WHO BUY IN. MCCARTHY HAS EVEN DRAGGED SOME heavy hitters in the health world down this rucking rabbit hole.

Later that night we found ourselves sitting around a dining room table, eating delivery Thai food with Peter and Amy Pollak. They're both heart doctors with the Mayo Clinic.

Amy is a preventative cardiologist who specializes in women's heart health. She has long red hair, speaks softly, and smiles constantly. She's the type of upbeat and disarming doctor who could calm the nerves of someone facing even the most dire bodily circumstances. Amy runs complicated medical tests to assess a patient's heart disease risk, then works with the patient to sidestep surgery by having them do all of the healthy stuff they've been avoiding for years. Exercising, eating better, destressing, etc.

"And if they don't listen to what I say, they get sent to Peter," said Amy. Peter is a heart surgeon who cuts people's chances of death by scalpel, stent, and other invasive measures. From the neck up he looks like a typical 40-something doctor. He has thinning gray hair, glasses, and is maybe even a little dorky. Neck down, he's built solid like McCarthy's Special Forces brothers.

The first doctor to prescribe exercise for health, around 600 BC, was Susruta, a physician in northern India. He noticed that his underactive patients seemed to be more disease prone. But "diseases fly from the presence of a person habituated to regular physical exercise," he said.

Early Greek physicians and philosophers believed exercise could warm, thin, and purge the body's unhealthy "humors." The physician to the Roman gladiators, Galen, believed that anything requiring "vigorous motion" and "labored breathing" would "'thin' the body, harden and strengthen muscles, increase flesh (muscle mass), and elevate blood volume while achieving 'good condition.'" This, he thought, would prevent and fix disease.

Just before the Industrial Revolution the world's first epidemiologist, an Italian doc named Bernardini Ramazzini, saw a link between jobs and disease. He noticed that people with active roles, like messengers who ran for their deliveries, experienced less sickness than people with sedentary jobs, like tailors and cobblers.

As the Industrial Revolution was altering the American way of life, the US Surgeon General's Office in 1915 released a report that highlighted the growing incidence of once rare diseases. Particularly heart disease. (The top killers had traditionally been pneumonia, tuberculosis, and diarrhea. Modern medicine was rendering these issues moot.)

The report noted that heart diseases seemed prevalent among people in stationary jobs. Five years later another report showed a correlation between the physical demands of a person's job and the age at which they'd die. More effortful work, it seemed, led to a longer life.

Yet these were mostly just smart observations. The scientific equivalent of "Hey, that's neat."

But after World War II a London-based epidemiologist named Jerry Morris was riding the bus and saw an opportunity for scientific rigor. London's double-decker bus drivers sat for about 90 percent of their workdays. The bus conductors, meanwhile, spent the day climbing the vehicles' stairs. Morris began systematically studying these men and their heart attack rates.

His work discovered that the conductors experienced 61 percent fewer heart attacks.

Scientists and doctors are still learning just how powerful exercise is. The NIH recently dumped $170 million into a research project called MoTrPAC (Molecular Transducers of Physical Activity Consortium). "I think we're going to find a whole host of new things we don't know about exercise," a team leader on the MoTrPAC project told me.

"Most of my patients just need to be more active," said Amy. "It's plain and simple." They're oftentimes people who aren't exactly in peak physical condition. And the addition of exercise can, quite literally, work miracles.

The editor in chief of the *British Medical Journal,* Dr. Fiona Godlee, recently published a letter titled "The Miracle Cure." "As miracle cures are hard to come by," she wrote, "any claims that a treatment is 100 percent safe and effective must always be viewed with intense skepticism. There is perhaps one exception. Physical activity.

"People who are active have lower rates of cardiovascular disease, cancer, and depression," wrote Godlee. And "the science grows stronger by the day."

Amy spooned some green curry onto her plate and began talking about the relative merits of different types of exercise. "Walking is great. All my patients can walk," she said. "Then if the person walks with a pack with a little weight it'll increase the challenge and their heart rate."

The Pollaks are rucking converts because it takes an approachable exercise like walking and allows a person to increase the strain to their heart incrementally. This in turn dials up their cardio fitness. And the higher a person's cardio fitness, according to stacks of medical literature, the further that person is from nearly all of the popular ways humans now die.

Heart disease is the Jeffrey Dahmer of modern ailments. It kills more than 25 percent of us. That's one person in the United States dying of it every 37 seconds. Expanding fitness just a bit—the equivalent of a person improving their max running speed from five to six miles an hour—reduces the risk of heart disease by 30 percent, according to the American Heart Association.

Next is cancer. It kills 22.8 percent of us. The most fit people face a 45 percent lower risk of dying from the disease, according to a study in the *Annals of Oncology.*

Then we have accidents. They take 6.8 percent of us. If a person is in a serious car accident, being in shape drops their chances of dying by 80 percent, according to a study in the *Emergency Medical Journal.* If the docs have to operate—regardless of whether it's an emergency or a planned surgery—fitter people also face fewer surgical complications and recover faster than unfit people, say scientists in Brazil.

Lung disease gets 5.3 percent of us. Fitter people have lungs that are 2.8 times less at risk of disease, say scientists at Northwestern University. The recent pandemic Covid-19 attacked the lungs and could cause pneumonia and, in turn, death. A study in *Annals of Epidemiology* found that fitter people face a smaller risk of developing pneumonia compared to the unfit. And the CDC found that people infected with Covid-19 who also suffered from preventable lifestyle diseases driven by a lack of fitness were six times more likely to be hospitalized.

Keep descending the death list: stroke, diabetes, Alzheimer's, and so on. Fitness fends off most maladies. Being out of shape is the new smoking, only worse. Research suggests that smoking takes 10 years off a person's life, while the combined effects of being unfit may take as many as 23.

Research from the National Cancer Institute and Johns Hopkins suggests that the more a person marinates in exercise-induced discomfort, the more death resistant they'll be. A massive study discovered that for every small increase in fitness, a person's risk of keeling over drops by 15 percent.

There is, in fact, no such thing as "too much" exercise. The Johns Hopkins scientists found that people who exercised more than three to five times the amount the government recommends were radically less likely to die. That's between 450 and 750 minutes, or 7 and 12 hours a week.

Many people think that too much exercise can cause heart attacks. But there was also no excess risk posed by exercising even ten times the amount the government recommends, equivalent to 25 hours a week. The Hadza exercise about that much and show "no evidence of risk factors for cardiovascular disease," wrote Raichlen in a study.

Life for nearly all of time used to give us a daily dose of this weekly 450-minute medicine. Until our mass transition into the built environment, in front of screens and behind desks, cut off our supply. Meanwhile, a swell of exercise evidence is causing more doctors to believe that getting closer to our ancestral activity trends is not only a hedge against sickness but also a cure for it.

"Have you heard of the CLEVER study?" asked Peter Pollak. It is, apparently, a piece of research that cardiology nerds clamor over. (CLEVER stands for Claudication: Exercise Vs. Endoluminal Revascularization.)

It studied the effect of two treatments for artery claudication, a common and growing problem among inactive people in which the leg arteries become clogged with fatty plaque. The condition causes pain, increases the risk of a stroke or heart attack, and can lead a person to stop walking. At which point the person's quality of life plummets while their risk of death skyrockets, according to scientists in Norway.

In the study, one group had a surgical stent inserted into their backed-up artery. The other group walked for an hour three times a week. The docs then followed up with the patients after 6 and 18 months.

Surgery is, of course, convenient. Show up. Go under. Wake fixed.

But Peter would rather not cut into a person unless it's absolutely necessary. Because surgery also comes with risks of complications that can make matters worse, and it typically doesn't fix the underlying issue causing the problem. If exercise could do the same as surgery, that would be a hell of a lot safer and cheaper deal.

"The two groups showed basically no difference," said Peter. Both groups had equal reductions in pain. Both could walk easier and more frequently.

"They didn't measure this," said Peter, "but the exercise group was probably better off because exercise provides benefits far beyond the artery condition." Exercise helped their other arteries, fought back cancer, made them more robust and slightly better looking when naked, etc.

Movement also beats some medications, according to research published in the *New England Journal of Medicine*. The scientists took a group of people who were about to develop type-2 diabetes. One group received Metformin, the most common drug used to prevent, delay, and treat diabetes. Another group exercised just 15 minutes per day.

"I was a consultant for the physical activity intervention arm of the study. I remember being very disappointed," said Wendy Kohrt, PhD, a researcher with the NIH who was involved in the study. "I thought the bar had been set too low for the level of exercise."

The scientists followed up after three years. "The exercise intervention was not only as effective, it was *more* effective," said Kohrt. The pill poppers reduced their incidence of diabetes by 31 percent. Not bad. Except when compared to the exercise group. They dropped their diabetes incidence by 58 percent. Exercise was nearly twice as effective. "So I think that's the study that showed the potential therapeutic benefit of doing things that don't involve taking pills," she said.

Exercise isn't medication for every ailment, of course. But it's often more effective in treating strokes and relieving depression. Exercise and antidepressants lead to similar brain changes. Both grow the hippocampus, a section of the brain that is often shrunken in depressed people. Which is why the American Psychological Association now suggests that psychiatrists prescribe exercise.

"In the veteran space there's so much talk of mental health, but no talk of physical health," said McCarthy. "Good things can come if vets get out and get physically well. I mean, that's what did it for me."

"I also like that rucking requires an element of strength," said Peter. He points out that it engages more muscles than a walk or a run. "Muscles are thirsty. More muscle demands more blood, which means your heart has to work harder."

The strength research is just like the cardio research. The stronger a person is, the less likely they are to croak. Some scientists believe strong muscles are more important than strong lungs.

"Muscle causes, controls, and regulates your ability to move. If you lose muscle quality and can't move, everything else fails quickly." That's according to Andy Galpin, PhD, who runs the Biochemistry and Molecular Exercise Physiology Laboratory at California State–Fullerton and conducts research for NASA.

Swedish research found that the strongest among a massive group of men of all ages were the least likely to die over two decades. The effect held even when the researchers removed any cardiovascular benefits from strength training. Other research shows that healthy muscle controls blood sugar levels and mitigates inflammation. That condition is something of a pervasive killer, implicated in pretty much all the diseases that end modern people.

Another data set of nearly 2 million healthy people showed that those with the strongest grip and leg strength were 31 and 14 percent less likely to die over two decades.

Nearly all researchers agree that strength and cardio can't be an either/or proposition. "Endurance exercise is not muscle building, and it probably isn't even muscle maintaining," said Kohrt. She served on the federal advisory committee that wrote the report the physical activity guidelines are based on. "This is why we recommended in addition to a hundred and fifty minutes a week of endurance exercise that people also do resistance exercise to build and maintain muscle mass."

"Rucking is particularly great for women for this reason," said Emily McCarthy, Jason's wife, who was also at dinner at the Pollaks'. She's a former CIA operative who now co-runs GORUCK. "You can build strength without having to go lift at a gym."

"And it also won't increase our patients' injury risk like running could," added Amy. Carrying seems to take the average person and toughen them. Stronger heart and muscles. More resilient joints.

McCarthy recently traveled to the University of Waterloo, where he met with Dr. Stuart McGill. McGill is a leading authority on fitness and back health. "It's no coincidence that the militaries of the world have chosen rucking as the tool to create that physical and mental fusion of toughness," McGill told McCarthy. "You can push someone and really give them a little bit of toughness exposure without high risk of injury."

One analysis found that "27% to 70% of recreational and competitive distance runners sustain an overuse running injury during any 1-year period." Our inactivity seems to mess up our movement patterns and cause muscular imbalances. These often lead to injury when people start pounding the pavement.

Scientists at the University of Pittsburgh, for example, investigated what activities most often injure Special Forces soldiers. Running was the top offender. It caused six times more injuries than rucking.

Take the knees. A study in the journal *Medicine and Science in Sports and Exercise* found running hits the knees with forces 8 times greater than body weight per stride. The same figure for walking is about 2.7. So, in practice, this means that with each running stride a 175-pound person loads their knees with about 1,400 pounds. For walking the figure is about 470.

And despite the initial promises of minimalist and barefoot running, the method for most doesn't seem to be any less injurious than running in traditional shoes, according to a review of all the research published in the scientific journal *Sports Health*.* "There's a reason they call it 'runner's knee,'" said McCarthy.

---

* This is likely explained by a variety of factors. Westerners often transition to barefoot/ minimal running too quickly. They also practice the method on paved roads, and are on average heavier people. Generally, people in developing countries who run barefoot for tens of miles with seemingly less injury (like the Tarahumara in *Born to Run*) (1) have been running that way since childhood; (2) run on softer earth; (3) have a lower body weight.

He consulted with University of Virginia scientists to learn the equivalent knee loads for rucking. If that same person wears a 30-pound ruck, the forces to the knee jump to about 555 pounds each step.*

That figure isn't insignificant. But it's roughly a third of the number for running. And it delivers equivalent cardio benefits, according to researchers at the University of South Carolina.

Walking's injury rate is roughly 1 percent. The figure climbs as a person loads a pack. But the risk is comparatively negligible at loads below 50 pounds, according to studies from the British and US militaries. (People who weigh less than 150 pounds may want to use less than 50 pounds, though.)

"The weight in the ruck is also a great equalizer, which also makes it more social," McCarthy said. "I ruck with my mom all the time. She takes ten pounds. I take fifty. We go the same speed but get the same effect. Outdoor physical activity with people—that's foundational. That's what *Homo sapiens* evolved to do, and it makes us happy."

Humans evolved doing physical work with friends, and sociality is deeply intertwined with effort. Being social while actively hunting and gathering improved our success and survival, according to research in *Nature*. Even today people are more likely to stick with more social exercise routines, says a study in *Frontiers in Psychology*.

The Pollaks and McCarthys ruck together often. They load their rucks, herd the kids, leash their dogs, and walk and catch up. There are also group rucks each Wednesday at GORUCK HQ. Sometimes more than 50 people from the Jacksonville area show up.

"It's so easy to integrate rucking into what you're already doing," said Emily. Ruck in to work. Or to dinner or the coffee shop. Or to the grocery store with a light pack and a food-filled one on the way home. "We've drifted into viewing exercise as a 30-minute class we do at a gym or on a machine alone in front of a screen," said McCarthy.

---

* The math is 175 + 30 x 2.7.

Raichlen agreed with this notion. When we spoke he directed me to a viral photo that showed a group of people taking the escalator rather than the stairs to get to an L.A.-based gym. "The photo is a microcosm of how we think about exercise," Raichlen told me. "It's this half-hour bout and then we sit around the rest of the day."

"When people are like 'Must be nice to have those genes,' my response is 'Show me your phone,'" said McCarthy. "They inevitably have like four thousand steps for the day. People just need to be more active generally. I don't really care if it's rucking or not. I just think rucking is approachable for everyone and offers many benefits."

"But you do sell rucks," I said. "Are people ever skeptical of your intentions?"

"Sure, we sell rucks," replied McCarthy. "But this is America and we believe in the role of businesses to drive social and societal change. We want people to get out and be active together. Doing more of that is how we define success. Not by the amount of rucks that sit in anyone's closet, but by how many people are out using them."

He continued. "Look, we're not inventing anything new here. Man has been carrying since we stood upright and freed our hands. We're just promoting something that is simple and has worked for our species since the very beginning."

I thought of a point Galpin made to me: "If I said, 'Hey, we're going for a two-hour hike. Or we're going to dead-lift at body weight. Or do some grappling or kickboxing today,' and that gives you anxiety, that's a big problem. I'm not saying those things shouldn't be challenging. But you should be able to do pretty much any physical activity well." In our pursuit of better living we've allowed comfort to calcify our natural movements and strengths. Without conscious discomfort and purposeful exercise—a forceful push against comfort creep—we'll only continue to become weaker and sicker.

21

80 PERCENT

DONNIE REACHES THE teepee first. He dumps his pack, which lands with a slumping thud. William arrives and throws down his own bag as Donnie takes a long drag from his aluminum water bottle.

I reach the two and remove one of my pack's shoulder straps, then carefully sling the weight to my side. William steps forward to help me set the pack back-side down so the antlers reach into the sky.

I then wander off in a daze and find a soft moss patch to fall into. It's starting to snow.

Forget runner's high. This is carrier's high. Endorphins are coursing through my veins and the absence of weight makes me feel like I'm levitating above the tundra. My energy is long gone, legs feel completely blown, and shoulders and torso are mostly numb. So I melt into the moss and marinate in those feel-good chemicals as snowflakes touch my face.

But only for a moment.

"Steaks, boys?" William says. I tip up my head. He's rifling through the big bag of meat. His bare hand emerges gripping an 18-inch cylinder of dark flesh.

I'm up. The more than ten hours of physical work—five of them unlike any I've done in my life—have shut off my ability to process any higher-order thoughts or concepts. But my zombie brain instinctively responds to the notion of meat and replacing all those spent calories.

In the teepee I fire up the stove while William works his knife against the caribou backstrap. He cuts inch-thick steaks, then slices them further into bite-size medallions.

"Look what I got . . . ," Donnie sings. He's holding an onion and "this wicked game seasoning I brought from home." Delicious contraband he carried so many miles just for this moment.

Williams sees this and makes the sound a child might when her parents announce that the family is going out for ice cream. It's an *oooo-weee* noise that falls somewhere between toddler and piglet.

Donnie flips open a knife and begins bisecting the onion and peeling its leaves. The onion sizzles in the pan as William continues to butcher.

The ruby chunks of meat fall into the pan with a crackle. William hits them with the seasoning, and the sound and smell of dinner fills the teepee. Outside the snow is thickening and moistening the air. Our exhales are thick clouds.

"Well," says Donnie as he looks at me. "Your bull. You get the first bite."

William stabs his knife into the pan and then thrusts a medallion at me. It singes my fingers as I pull it from the knife. I bite in.

It's soft like prime rib, but richer and leaner. Perfectly seasoned. It's better than any meat I've ever tasted.

Sure, in a blind taste test against the top offering from the finest New York City steakhouse this meat probably wouldn't win. But food enjoyment is context dependent. Research shows that the exact same dish can taste better or worse depending on a variety of factors. Like where a person is eating it, who they're eating it with, how hungry they are, and, apparently, how hard they worked for it.

We each eat a Mountain House dinner and share about three pounds of meat among us. The stove is eventually shut off and the teepee grows even colder. We all burrow into our sleeping bags.

Donnie mentions that the smell of the meat "will probably definitely" attract grizzlies tonight. I tell him the story my high school geometry teacher told the class about the grizzly slapping off the young deckhand's head.

"Probably bullshit," he says. Then we're all silent.

I'm utterly worn. Previously untested areas of my back, butt, shoulders, sides, front, etc., all feel awake after a decades-long slumber. But I'm also not broken down. Nothing hurts. It's a satisfying feeling of exhaustion.

The Arctic has forced me into what you might call fundamental movements and body position. I carry weight everywhere. When I sit it's ass to hardpack, squatting, or flailed out on frosty, rocky ground, with stones pressing into my muscles. While glassing I can't sit in one position for even 15 minutes, much less 8 hours. I'm constantly shifting as the hard earth starts to hurt me.

When we've stalked animals it's all contorted and waddle-walking across hundreds of yards. Or we've lain belly down in the dirt and dragged ourselves. Even sleep happens at odd angles, and my thin pad forces me to twist and turn at night.

These movements and positions are unyielding out here. And they've mostly all been engineered out of modern life.

"So many people who work out chase infinite cardio or strength capacity," Kelly Starrett, a doctor of physical therapy who consults for various professional sports teams, told me. "People need just as much movement capacity. Many people go months without taking their joints through a full range of motion. People are de-evolving."

Consider a day of the average American office worker. He wakes up on a pillow-topped, waist-high mattress, then slides his legs onto the floor. He shuffles around the house a bit, then moves into a car seat to commute. Once he arrives at the office he sits in an office chair, which has a slew of dials and switches, all of which are designed to offer ecstasy-inducing ergonomics. After sitting at work, the man is back sitting in his car. When he gets home, he sits at a table for dinner, then on the couch for TV. Then it's back into the horizontal position for bed. Repeat until retirement.

Katy Bowman, a biomechanist, told me that many bodies today suffer from "diseases of captivity." She compared modern humans to captive killer whales. "Orcas in captivity often have fins that flop over," she said. "In the natural world this isn't an issue. The fin has enough loading from swimming a hundred miles every day to keep it upright."

A human body's ideal loading was our daily doses of carrying, walking, running, squatting, digging, and more. Instead of flopped fins, our outcome is poor movement, pain, and chronic diseases.

And a person's movement is only as bad as they've made it, said Bowman. Kids have full command of their joints and can easily squat, lunge, lift overhead, and more. But movement is a use-it-or-lose-it proposition. Those kids eventually sit at school desks, then join average Americans behind a work desk. But, as Mayo Clinic researchers put it, "The human, simply put, was not designed to sit all day."

But through movement we bloom. Research suggests that moving through full ranges of natural motion may jump-start dormant cells that fight aging. Conversely, a lack of complete movement can potentially cause cellular maladaptations, making people more likely to age poorly, according to a study in *Medicine & Science in Sports & Exercise*.

Rediscovering lost movement, a swell of research is showing, can fix one of the most insidious diseases of captivity: back pain (to take just one example).

About 80 percent of Americans will experience back pain sometime in their life. A quarter of people say they've had it in the last few months. It's the most common place people experience pain, and the most frequent reason people see a doctor or take a sick day from work. Back pain costs our economy $100 billion every year.

Back pain sometimes comes from something a doctor can scan, see on an image, and diagnose. Like an injured disk, tumor, osteoporosis, or fracture. But 85 percent of it is labeled "nonspecific," which is unseeable pain that appears from the ether. Scientists at Harvard estimate that 97 percent of this nonspecific back pain is caused by the way we now live. By captivity in our modern environment.

When I met with the anthropologist Daniel Lieberman he explained to me that much of this peculiar back pain exists on a U-shaped curve.

Picture a graph that shows pain on the *y* axis and activity level on the *x* axis. The data will be shaped like a U. This means that the groups with the most pain are both the least and most active. The people with the least amount of pain are at the bottom of the U and they have a medium activity level. Case in point, Lieberman said, is that studies show that people who perform what we think of as "backbreaking work" experience roughly the same amount of back pain compared to office workers. For example, 38 percent of farmers in northern China experienced back pain over a handful of months, while the number was anywhere from 33 to 46 percent among Chinese office workers. Research from Australia, meanwhile, discovered that people who do a broad range of physical activity are less likely to experience pain.

This may seem to suggest that too much activity is bad. But other data reveals the truth. Back pain from "too much" seems to be due to performing one physical activity at the expense of all others. "Probably from very weird, bizarre kinds of movements that people didn't do in the past," said Lieberman. "No one had to lift Amazon Prime boxes all day." Too little activity is quite a similar problem, except it's caused by a weird, bizarre *lack* of movement. A life of sitting, standing, and lying down.

"We used to be very active movement generalists," said Bowman. But we've now outsourced most of our movement to machines, chairs, soft beds, and more. When our work does require movement, it's often specific, repetitive, and destructive. "There are almost no remaining 'movement generalists' who are meeting their daily movement needs anymore," said Bowman.

Even our past inactive moments weren't entirely lazy. Research shows that hunter-gatherer tribes actually rest just as much as we do. Yet they don't seem to suffer from chronic back pain.

Lieberman explained to me that if I want to understand this phenomenon I should think about the difference between sitting in a La-Z-Boy recliner, a stool, and the squat position. "Chairs that have back rests require even less physical activity than, say, sitting on a stool or squatting, so they're even more comfortable," he said.

When we sit in our comfortable chairs, we don't so much sit as dissolve into their cushioning. Each of our muscles slackens like we've gone brain dead. "But our bodies aren't well adapted for chairs," said Lieberman.

David Raichlen ran a study where he tested how hunter-gatherers' resting positions influenced their muscle activity. They mostly squat or sit on the ground. "Squatting or sitting without their backs resting, unsurprisingly, increased their lower-back-muscle activation significantly," said Raichlen. Resting in a squat or kneeling lightly engages all the muscles in the lower body and torso. Sitting on a stool requires less work, but a person must still engage their core and back muscles to stay upright.

The takeaway: "Human physiology likely evolved in a context that included substantial inactivity, but increased muscle activity during sedentary time, suggesting an inactivity mismatch with the more common chair-sitting postures found in contemporary urban populations," Raichlen wrote in the study. This theory is called the inactivity mismatch hypothesis.

Our comfortable, supportive-to-the-extreme chairs, couches, and beds of today do the work that our muscles are meant to. And muscle is use-it-or-lose-it stuff. Just ten days of not using a muscle significantly weakens and shrinks it.

Then when chair-weakened people bend over to lift something or move into a new position, their body is brittle. It breaks. And this is likely a critical reason why back pain is so common in the most comfortable societies and essentially absent among movement generalists. Populations in Asia and the Middle East who rest and do many activities in the squatting position, for example, see little to no hip and lower-back issues.

When our modern pain arises, we don't listen to what it's trying to tell us. Pain was and still is an evolutionary advantage. It's our brain's way of telling us we're doing something potentially dangerous. A warning of harm and threat. A use of discomfort to suggest a change that will improve our health and safety. Yet we mute it with pills, surgery, or rest. Those are easy treatments, but evidence shows they're usually not a solution. "Rest, opioids, spinal injections, and surgery . . . will not reduce back-related disability or its long-term consequences," wrote a global team of 12 doctors and scientists who studied all the evidence on back pain treatment.

Back pain is one of the leading reasons for opioid prescriptions. Yet the scientists found that pills only temporarily mute pain and don't work over the long term. For more relief, people must keep popping more, stronger pills. This leads to addiction in 20 percent of patients. Treating back pain with powerful painkillers was, in fact, a key driver of the opioid epidemic, according to the research.

Then there's surgery. Forget the cost. Researchers at the University of Cincinnati Medical School tracked roughly 1,500 workers who had debilitating back pain that was keeping them from work. Half of the workers had surgery and half did not. After two years, 75 percent of those who had surgery were still in excruciating pain and unable to return to work. But 67 percent of those who *didn't* have surgery were working again. Of the people who went under the knife, 36 percent had complications, 27 percent required another surgery, and the whole group had higher rates of opioid use.

"But people now become slaves to their computer and think, 'Oh, I just have to exercise. I'll just go blast in the gym for forty-five minutes,'" said Dr. McGill, the back health and fitness expert. "That's a problem in terms of intensity and workload—people cross a biological tipping point." His work shows that people who sit all day then attack the gym have higher rates of back dysfunction compared to couch potatoes. "Unfair, I know," he said.

"A much more healthful recipe would be more gentle exercise throughout the day," said McGill. Running the body through all the movements it can do: squat, lunge, plank, hinge, hang, twist, carry, bend, and more. Raichlen's study backs up the health of resting in a squatting or kneeling position over lounging in a chair.

Or adding carrying into our daily routines. Rucking was found not only to have no association with low back pain, it even helped prevent it. The weight pulls people out of the slumped-over position that's so common among desk workers. And it engages all the core muscles and glute muscles. Strong core and glutes, which become particularly weakened through too much sitting, are two of the best defenses against back pain, according to the Cleveland Clinic and Bowman.

McGill said carrying forces a person to stand tall and lock down the muscles that protect their spine. McGill, for example, used the suitcase carry exercise—carrying a weight at one side while walking and keeping the torso vertical—to rehabilitate the dysfunctional spine of a champion powerlifter.

"That's a wonderful exercise," he said. And it can be practiced anytime.

THE TEEPEE IS BRIGHT WHEN I WAKE. DONNIE RUSTLES AS HE HEARS ME UNZIP MY sleeping bag.

"What time is it?" he asks.

"Nine a.m."

We'd slept for almost 12 hours. William is still out. So we silently brew coffee and take it outside. The steam from my cup fogs my eyes as I sip while surveying the scene. Snow coats the ground and mountains around us. A quarter moon still hangs on the horizon. The only sound is the faint trickling of a distant stream.

We recount everything that happened yesterday. The moment that bull crested the knoll. When we both noticed his limp. How his weathered body and elaborate antlers showed what a storied life he had lived out here.

"I would love to know how he got that limp," Donnie says. "I'd guess from fighting. But you never know. And that scene where you shot. With The Fort behind us. It was spectacular, just spectacular."

I tell him I still can't get over how taxing the packing out was.

"You learn a lot about yourself and how you're built out here," he says. "William and I were talking about how you've done better than we anticipated."

I don't know whether that's a compliment of my abilities or an inadvertent dig. So I just drink my coffee.

Donnie realizes this. "Oh . . . no. It's just . . . no one understands how challenging this all is. [Hunting] guide friends of mine tell me all the time about clients who train in the gym year-round for a hunt and then get out in the wild and quit on the first or second day. Or they'll offer the guide a massive tip to carry out all the meat. This experience can't be replicated in a gym."

William emerges from the tent. His long hair is a rat's nest and he's wearing long johns and untied boots.

"We need more fuckin' water," he says.

The work continues. I grab a jug, then begin hiking the half mile down to a half-frozen stream.

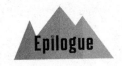

81.2 YEARS

WE TREKKED AND hunted through Alaska for another couple weeks, experiencing plenty more misogi-like challenges I could never have had in a tamed world. We hiked steeper and longer hills and faced worsening weather. We observed grizzlies as they lumbered through the valley—one came into our camp at night and savaged my caribou's hide, which we'd laid out to dry. We even had a fox take up semi-permanent residence at our campsite. He'd circle the teepee, make eyes at us, and steal the caribou trimmings we'd toss into nearby bushes. Then he'd hang around, waiting for more. Donnie also successfully hunted an old caribou. His antlers were wide and high, like goalposts, and his body was beat all to hell.

Then early one morning Brian messaged Donnie on his emergency GPS device. A serious storm was rolling in. Big blizzards and savage winds, the type that could prevent a plane from landing for a long time. We didn't want to push this Alaska voyage past five weeks.

"Looks like we'll pack up and be out of here early tomorrow, boys," Donnie said.

That day we experienced a full caribou migration. Imagine thousands of animals converging at once, like ants swarming a hill. "I've been to Alaska for months at a time for nearly thirty years in a row,"

Donnie said. "And I've never seen anything like this. Awe is the only word for it."

I exited the teepee that night to experience the cold and silence one last time. The sun was nearly down, darkening the skeletons of the willows as it illuminated their leaves. The clouds were long and gray and moving south just like the caribou.

Brian and Mike touched down along a rocky point of the sliver-shaped island the next morning. We'd spent a week there among grizzly tracks and the carcasses of the dog salmon the bears had ripped apart. My return to the tamed world began.

BACK AT THE RAM AVIATION CONEX BOX, I GORGED MYSELF ON FRESH FOOD, EATING four apples and an entire bag of carrots. My seatmates on the return flight from Kotzebue to Anchorage—two other hunters who'd each been out for four nights—responded with a blend of astonishment and skepticism when I told them how long we'd spent in the Arctic. "A MONTH???" one said. I nodded. He just stared at me awkwardly, so I asked, "Are you going to eat those peanuts?"

I entered the hotel in Anchorage looking like a cast member from some post-apocalyptic movie. Face weather burned and fully bearded. Body callused, bruised, cut, hardened, and ten pounds leaner. My pack and pants were stained red in places by caribou blood. I was entirely filthy and smelled like a feed lot blended with a salmon run.

I'd spent the last month sitting in the dirt, sleeping in the dirt, and shitting in the dirt. I'd buried my hands in the innards of dead animals and carried their organs barehanded across the land. I'd pissed all over myself when erratic wind pushed my urine back onto my long johns. I'd even succumbed in fits of boredom to dissecting clods of bear poop. And then I ate breakfast, lunch, and dinner with those hands.

There hadn't been a sink, shower, bar of soap, or Purell pump within miles up there, and so I'd rinsed my hands with snow or river water. That same unpurified water hydrated me. I was dirty from the inside out.

And so it was that my first act upon entering my hotel room was to turn the shower on to full blast and then strip down and purge the film of gunk that coated my skin and clogged every pore and crevice. As I lathered and re-lathered, I eyed the pile of gnarly clothes on the bathroom floor, thinking I should burn it for the good of humanity.

But a new body of research is showing that I may have actually done more harm than good by sanitizing all that natural bacteria from my body.

Stephanie Schnorr is an anthropologist at the University of Nevada, Las Vegas. I first met her before leaving for Alaska. She studies the feces from forgotten tribes to better understand the human microbiome.

It's not the sexiest of research, but she's something of a world expert on the 4.5 pounds of germs, bacteria, fungi, protozoa, and viruses that live on and in you, and what they do for your health. It's a field that took off only a couple of decades ago. But researchers like Schnorr have since determined that your microbiome is almost a separate organ keeping you alive and well from head to toe.

Schnorr has an office at an evolutionary research institute in Austria and one at UNLV. But the core of her research takes place in the East African Rift Valley, around the shores of salty Lake Eyasi in northwestern Tanzania.

"Have you ever been to West Texas?" she asked me as we sat across from each other in a hygienic Las Vegas coffee shop. "Where the Hadza live is a lot like West Texas. Dry. Lots of rocks and scrubby trees."

Schnorr lived among the tribe in 2013. She watched as its members foraged for wild plants, bugs, and tubers that "look like a bark-covered stick." Or while they hunted for baboons, birds, antelope, and wildebeests. "They'll wait in a blind by a watering hole at night," said Schnorr. "Then they ambush and shoot poison arrows. The poison is usually a tar they make from the desert rose plant."

They carry all that food back to camp and eat it while sitting in the dirt. Sometimes that food is cooked. Other times it's raw. They're outside always. The Hadza also bathe and wash their hands, rarely, in muddy, sometimes manure-filled puddles. They shit outside. Probably have gotten piss on themselves, too.

This lifestyle might seem like a quick path to a deathly infection. But the Hadza are seemingly impervious to some of the diseases that take down many of us Westerners. They don't seem to get Crohn's, colitis, IBD, or even colon cancer. The first three diseases have been increasing rapidly in the developed world, and are now spreading into developing countries as they westernize.

Doctors are particularly concerned about the rise of colon cancer. It's already the third-most-common cancer. But it's increasingly becoming a cancer of young, otherwise-healthy people. A person born in 1990, for example, has double the risk of colon cancer and quadruple the risk of rectal cancer compared to someone born in 1950. Scientists at the University of Texas, Austin's MD Anderson Cancer Center project that colon cancer will rise by 90 percent among 20- to 34-year-olds over the next decade. A young person's risk is still low. But younger people are more likely to die from the disease, because it's often too far advanced by the time docs catch it.

There may be an answer. Studies around an emerging theory called the hygiene hypothesis have strongly linked the rise in these diseases and others to our supersanitized lives. Even mood, metabolism, and immunity are affected.

The West began its all-out war on germs in the 1800s. This is when we realized that some germs are the source of infectious disease. This battle has saved many lives and raged ever since. But it's also had some unintended consequences.

"We have this notion that germs cause disease. But we've given this blanket term of 'germs' to all microorganisms and think that we should therefore kill them all," said Schnorr. "We've dramatically increased the ways we sanitize our life. We sterilize the surfaces we come in contact with. We sterilize all our food by washing it excessively and then cooking it. We sterilize ourselves because we bathe all the time. We use antibiotics so we sterilize the inside of our body. We avoid getting dirty outside. So this means we now have far less exposure to *all* microorganisms."

Except not all germs or microorganisms are bad. The vast, vast majority are benign and many are beneficial. In fact, Harvard anthropologist Christina Warriner points out that there are more bacteria in the gut than stars in the galaxy. And scientists estimate that fewer than 100 of these species could hurt your health.

As we evolved we developed a mutually beneficial alliance with many of these microscopic living organisms. We gave them a home and they built our immune system and stress tolerance, helping us avoid sickness and become more robust and resilient. This is no revolutionary idea. It's exactly how vaccines work. Our bodies build immunity by experiencing an imitation of a bug.

Our constant, low-level exposures to a wide variety of microorganisms in the natural world toughened us. But we've since gone scorched earth on those organisms and removed ourselves from the environments where we'd experience them. Without exposure, our bodies may be more disease prone, seem to have a harder time fighting formerly powerless microbes, and even mistake the benign ones for bad guys, said Schnorr.

With that in mind, she found herself in East Africa. Schnorr wanted to know what the microbes living inside the guts of the "unhygienic" Hadza look like compared to those of "hygienic" Westerners. This might tell us something about what all this sanitization is doing to us.

The best way to measure gut bacteria is to analyze fecal samples. Which is to say that Schnorr needed the tribe members to shit in and return disposable containers she bought at Whole Foods.

"I gave them my pitch and they were all totally unmoved," she said. "And then one of the older men goes, 'We normally give it to the ground. But we'll give it to her.'"

The results from the samples were "a real shock," said Schnorr. The Hadza guts harbored a bacterium scientists then considered a "bad," "disruptor" bacterium. But, paradoxically, the Hadza are in many ways far healthier than "clean" Westerners.

"The Hadza microbiome shows a direct connection with their environment, and they benefit from that connection," said Schnorr. "They are much more robust, they get sick less, and basically don't get noncommunicable diseases."

The results of her study rocked the microbiology community, making the field rethink what they consider "good" and "bad" bacteria.

She said our sanitary lives, on the other hand, factor into our massive rates of chronic disease. "We sterilize everything. And here we are, more sick, fragile, and depleted," she said. "We've reduced the effectiveness of our immune system in determining what's actually harmful to us and what's not," she said. That can lead our systems to go "haywire."

Haywire systems do strange things. For example, they can mount massive defenses against foods that should be safe for us—like peanuts. Food allergies disproportionately affect people in the most sanitary nations. Ten percent of one-year-olds now suffer some degree of peanut allergy, and hospitalizations by peanut doubled over the last decade.

She compared our hygienic microbiomes to having "weaker armor." "So our health gets perturbed much more easily, and we're in a physiological state that's more likely to induce illness and cause harm. It's small, subtle, and chronic, pushing us in the direction of sickness," she said.

Meanwhile, people who haven't lived their life sanitized are tougher. "Maybe that person can sustain a few more hits to their health and not be as susceptible to disease," said Schnorr. "Or maybe they're more responsive to therapies and bounce back quicker if they get sick."

Our lack of exposure seems to put us in a state of chronic

inflammation, according to scientists at University College London. "[In the] USA and other high-income countries," wrote the researchers, "there is often constant low-grade inflammation which tends to be stable across individuals . . . in the absence of any clinically apparent inflammatory stimulus."

Then we throw "a lifetime of stress and sleep deprivation compounded with a poor diet and low activity and it seems to bring on chronic disease rather quickly," said Schnorr. Scientists at Northwestern University wrote, "All major diseases, including cardiovascular disease, diabetes, neurodegenerative disorders, arthritis, and cancers involve chronic inflammation."

"I mean, it's not like we're all walking around on the verge of death," said Schnorr. "There are *plenty* of healthy people in Western industrial societies. But I think on average we're more susceptible to chronic diseases." Microbes are also not the single ingredient of Hadza health—but they're surely a factor. A lack of exposure has even been linked to worse-off mental health, because some bacteria could produce substances that alter nerve cells.

Unfortunately, there's no pill that can alter our gut microbiomes to be more Hadza-like. "Because they take in microbes from food they pull from the dirt, as well as air and land," said Schnorr. "You really need continuous exposure to outside microbes." University of Chicago microbiome scientists have in fact declared that "dirt is good." The more time a person spends outside getting down and dirty in it, the better.

Diet is also critical, according to those London-based scientists. It "needs to be diverse and contain fiber and polyphenols found in plant products. A diet deficient in fiber can lead to progressive extinctions of important groups of [microbial] organisms," they wrote.

The shelves of modern grocery stores are filled with thousands upon thousands of things to eat. But research shows that most Americans consume a limited variety of foods. Our most commonly eaten foods, for example, are made mostly of refined flour, which has the fiber stripped from it. But a study of the Hadza, for example, found that they eat more than 600 foods, 70 percent of them unprocessed, fiber-filled plants.

"I eat a lot of organic plants," said Schnorr. "I eat many of them raw." Cooking not only kills microbes, it can also slightly lower fiber counts. Which isn't to say a person should eat every vegetable raw—the nutrients in some vegetables like tomatoes, carrots, and cabbage are more easily absorbed by our bodies after cooking—but we might benefit from not cooking *every* vegetable.

"It's also wise to avoid taking antibiotics unless absolutely necessary," said Schnorr. Antibiotics can be lifesaving. But in killing infection they also raze our gut microbiome. The CDC reports that at least 47 million antibiotic prescriptions in the United States are unnecessary. And this, the scientists say, "put[s] patients at needless risk for allergic reactions or the sometimes deadly diarrhea, *Clostridium difficile.*"

The CDC is also increasingly concerned that overprescription is allowing dangerous germs to evolve defenses against antibiotics. Because of this we may "lose the most powerful tool we have to fight life-threatening infections," stated the CDC's director. "Losing these antibiotics would undermine our ability to treat patients with deadly infections and cancer, provide organ transplants, and save victims of burns and trauma."

In the absence of an outbreak like Covid-19, where even Schnorr had no choice but to be belligerent with the Purell, she generally doesn't disinfect her home or hands. "I abhor sanitizer," she said. "And, trust me, you're going to survive if you don't shower. In fact, it can be beneficial." Harvard Medical School stated that a daily shower with antibacterial soap "upsets the balance of microorganisms on the skin and encourages the emergence of hardier, less friendly organisms that are more resistant to antibiotics." And also, "frequent baths or showers throughout a lifetime may reduce the ability of the immune system to do its job."

THE HADZA AREN'T THE ONLY PEOPLE SHOWING US WHAT THE FUTURE OF DISCOM-
fort science may look like. Researchers have long studied groups
around the world for their "harder to kill" traits. The Ama, or sea
women, of Japan and Korea first came on the radar of the US Department of Defense in the 1960s as it was establishing the US Navy
SEALs. The women are a particularly interesting example of what
happens to humans who repeatedly expose themselves to uncomfortable environments.

My shower—30 minutes and scorching—provided something else
I hadn't experienced in a month: warmth. Constant climatic comfort
is something else we also may want to rethink.

Roughly two or three thousand years ago, women in the tiny fishing villages of Japan and Korea began diving into the cold waters of
the Japan Sea and Pacific Ocean. No wetsuits. No breathing contrap-
tions. The women would strip down to a loincloth, diving trunks, or
nothing at all. They'd row or swim to a spot where the ocean's rocky
bottom was 10 to 90 feet below, and dive, scouring the cold, clear
ocean depths.

After a minute or three, the woman's hand would emerge from
the surf and clasp the side of her boat. Then her other hand would
rise, dumping into the boat a bucket of edible sea treasures like ab-
alone, uni, mussels, or seaweed. In the summer the Ama worked
six- to ten-hour days on the chilly water, doing more than 150 daily
dives. From late fall to early spring, the ocean water dropped to just
50 degrees and the air temperatures could be just a couple degrees
above freezing. But the Ama dove anyway, constantly pushing their
limits to discover the knife edge of exposure.

Department of Defense research on the Ama showed they had less
incidence of 14 of the 16 illnesses the scientists studied. Compared
to their fellow villagers, the women were less likely to catch a cold, to
get heart disease, to get arthritis, to get liver or kidney diseases, and

so on. And the diseases they had were hazards of the job—like hearing loss due to the pressure of the ocean on their eardrums. Other researchers discovered that the Ama also had larger lung volumes, stronger muscles, and better endurance. Not surprising for breath-holding swimmers.

Findings on the Ama forced researchers to reconsider the rules of physiology. Humans lapse into hypothermia when their core temperature drops to 95 degrees or below. But the Ama's winter core temperatures averaged a physiology-bending 94.5 degrees.

The scientists also wondered how all that time in the cold impacted the Ama's metabolisms. A cold body, after all, ignites a complex network of calorie-burning internal furnaces to ensure that its organs don't become dangerously chilled. So they picked at random 20 Ama and 20 villagers and invited them into a makeshift lab to have their metabolic rates tested. The data showed that the Ama burned an additional 1,000 calories a day.

Thanks in large part to the Ama research, scientists now know what's driving their 1,000-calorie burn: brown fat.

Brown fat is a metabolically active tissue. Brown fat in the cold acts like a furnace that burns our white fat (the type we try to lose with diet and exercise) to generate heat. Working brown fat cranks through more calories than working our muscles and brain. Which is exactly why a team of scientists in the Netherlands think that getting comfortable with the cold can be an effective weight-control tactic.

The bad news, the scientists say, is that our creature comforts have rendered brown fat moot.

"In the past century several dramatic changes in the daily living circumstances in Western civilization have occurred, affecting health. For example, we are much better able to control our ambient temperature," wrote the scientists. "[We] lack exposure to varied ambient temperature [because we] cool and heat our dwellings for maximal comfort while minimizing our body energy expenditure necessary to control body temperature."

The scientists call this burning of energy "non-shivering thermo-genesis." Research shows it can elevate metabolism anywhere from a small percentage to 30 percent. Which is why the scientists write, "Similar to exercise training, we advocate temperature training. . . . More-frequent cold exposure alone will not save the world, but [it] is a serious factor to consider."

The cost of leveraging the power of brown fat is, of course, braving the cold. The upside is that we don't have to dive into a frigid ocean for hours at a time to see a substantial benefit.

The research shows that anyone can become cold acclimatized. I noticed this with William and Donnie. People who spend a lot of time in colder temperatures, scientists say, are less impacted by temperature extremes. We need a week or two of exposure to reach the point where we feel comfortable in the cold and begin optimizing our cold furnaces.

In winter, the scientists recommend people lower their thermostats by three to four degrees each week. This slowly pushes our comfort zone, allowing us to adapt without unnecessary suffering. Then we can stop once we're living in 64 degrees. Another study conducted by the NIH found that people who slept in rooms in the mid-60s saw a 10 percent increase in their metabolic activity. They also saw improvements in health markers like blood sugar levels. A person can go full-on Ama if they want, by taking ice baths. Some do (and, of course, dramatically Instagram it). But it seems like overkill, in light of the research.

Cedars-Sinai, Johns Hopkins, and other leading medical research institutions are even finding that extreme cold can help prevent severe brain damage and death after dangerous medical events. Doctors bring a cardiac arrest patient's body temperature down to between 89 and 93 degrees for roughly 24 hours. This sets off a cascade of events that protect a compromised brain, like lowering its demand for oxygen and energy, preventing neuronal cell death, and decreasing inflammation and harmful free radicals.

THE SHERPAS OF NEPAL ARE ANOTHER GROUP THAT IS FORCING SCIENTISTS TO RE-
think the limits of the human body and how it responds to extreme
environments.

Dr. Andrew Murray has spent thousands of hours trekking the
world's highest mountains. The views are nice. But as a physiologist,
he said he's always been more fascinated by the people carrying his
stuff. "You'll be huffing and puffing your way up what looks like a
fairly gentle slope, but you're held back by the low oxygen," he told
me. "Then a porter will breeze by you. He's maybe much older than
you, and he's carrying your bags and other people's bags, walking
like it's a stroll in the park."

The Sherpa, an ethnic group in eastern Nepal, are most famous
for this high-altitude fitness. Although the sport of mountaineering
was pioneered by Westerners, Sherpas hold the world record for the
most Everest ascents as well as the most summits without supplemental oxygen. They also hold the majority of speed summiting records. Pemba Dorje Sherpa climbed from Everest's South Base Camp
to its summit with supplemental oxygen in 8 hours and 10 minutes,
while Kazi Sherpa completed the feat without supplemental oxygen
in 20 hours and 24 minutes.

Murray recently conducted a study to see if Sherpa fitness was
solely from years of mountaineering, or if perhaps the extreme land
that the Sherpas come from had given them some sort of edge. The
existing data showed a paradox.

As the average person gains altitude, their body responds by pro-
ducing more oxygen-carrying red blood cells. Yet, curiously, previous
studies found that Sherpas do ramp up their red blood cell production when climbing, but not at nearly the rate of lowlanders. Which
means Sherpas actually register *less* oxygen in their blood than we do
while climbing.

To solve the mystery, Murray took thigh muscle biopsies on a group of Sherpas and Westerners at low altitudes. The groups—who were matched for age, sex, and general fitness level—then trekked from Katmandu to Everest Base Camp. Once they arrived at the 17,600-foot camp, the scientists took the same biological measurements.

The biopsies showed that at altitude the Sherpas' mitochondria—tiny power plants within human cells that power our bodies—produced more ATP, or energy, using less oxygen. They also found that the Sherpas used fat as fuel more efficiently.

"It's interesting because the Sherpas are actually unremarkable at sea level," said Murray. "You don't see them winning marathons. Their adaptation is not one that gives them super performance at sea level, but it does at altitude when the oxygen is scarce."

In other words, Westerners have the engine of a gas-guzzling SUV, while the Sherpas are more like a sensible hybrid that sips fuel. When fuel is abundant—at low altitude—both engines get the job done. But when you climb into a fuel-scarce, high-altitude environment, the more efficient engine is optimal. It helps the Sherpas climb farther, faster, and with less effort.

Even more striking, the team of scientists retook the measurements of both groups after they'd spent two months at Everest Base Camp. The findings showed that the energy levels in the muscles of the lowlanders dropped. Yet, like a flower exposed to the sun, the Sherpas' muscle energy levels bloomed, steadily increasing despite having less oxygen.

Murray published his results in *Proceedings of the National Academy of Sciences,* and said that Nepali Sherpas have evolved to perform like superhumans at altitude.

Murray's findings are an important first step in developing treatments for intensive-care-unit patients suffering from hypoxia, or a lack of oxygen. Hypoxia is life-threatening and occurs in healthy people at high altitude, and also in critical-care patients. Currently, doctors add oxygen to these patients' blood. But that thickens the blood and can cause complications like clogged blood vessels.

Murray's research is in its infancy, but the ultimate goal is to develop a method that allows patients to become more Sherpa-like and use what little oxygen they have more efficiently. This would lead to better health outcomes in sick people—and, perhaps, better performance in athletes.

We can experience similar benefits by living and training at altitude, according to an article in the scientific journal *Sports Medicine*. Endurance coaches since the 1960s have looked for a competitive edge by having their athletes "train high, race low," which ramps up oxygen-carrying red blood cell counts.

But the *Sports Medicine* research team found that altitude training does far more than that. It also leads to changes in mitochondria, which make our muscles more efficient, and improves how we buffer exercise-induced acids, allowing us to go harder longer. The catch is, a person can't just spend a weekend in the mountains and expect to emerge like a Sherpa. Prolonged, repeated bouts at altitude— mountain misogis, perhaps—lead to the most profound changes.

ONE OF THE MOST PROMISING ONGOING RESEARCH PROJECTS INTO THE FUTURE OF discomfort science is happening in Iceland. Shortly after I returned from Alaska, I traveled there to meet a man studying one of Earth's most hard-to-kill populations. He, in fact, is part of them.

I'd heard rumors of Dr. Kari Stefansson: In his 70s and built like an NFL tight end at six foot six and 220 pounds of raw muscle. One hundred percent Icelandic, with the white hair and blue eyes and everything you'd expect. Also brilliant.

Stefansson ran the Harvard neurology department for a while, until he left to open deCODE, a 190-scientist-strong genetic research company housed in a modern mega-laboratory in Reykjavik. The place holds more data than all of the country's banking system.

Stefansson and his team have sequenced the genotypes of 60 percent of living Icelanders, and their scientific studies have been cited about 200,000 times. This work has made Stefansson one of the richest men in Iceland and a national celebrity.

Stefansson is a great explorer of the human genome who is searching for information that could lead to treatments for many of the diseases that kill us. Iceland happens to be the perfect spot for his work.

Iceland is a lot like the Hotel California, in the sense that once people check in, they never leave. A handful of people arrived in Iceland about 1,100 years ago and populated the island, and few have come and gone since. The majority of Icelanders come from a single family tree. It's so common for Icelanders to have unknown cousins that the government created a genealogical dating app so people can avoid familial hookups.

For a geneticist like Stefansson, Iceland and its people are a scientific wellspring. With few people migrating in or out, there is less genetic variation among Icelanders. Therefore there is less confusing background noise in the data. The place offers a massive, naturally occurring control group.

This means that Stefansson and his team can more easily track diseases as they transfer through family lines. From there they can single out the genes that could lead people to get sick and die. The research done by deCODE has discovered genes—single bad actors among 3 billion—involved in heart disease, Alzheimer's, schizophrenia, and cancer.

But there's a flip side; deCODE has also found some genes that could cause humans to be well and live longer. And that's what Stefansson is really interested in. He found in the APP gene a variant that offers complete protection against age-related mental decline and Alzheimer's disease. And a variant in the ASGR1 gene that gives its holders significant protection from heart disease. He's found other variants that greatly reduce the risk of developing diabetes and prostate cancer.

Stefansson has also come to believe that there might be another gene lurking within Icelanders that makes them tougher than the rest of us.

The World Health Organization recently discovered that Icelandic men are the longest living on Earth. Guys from Iceland rack up roughly 81.2 years. That's 13.2 more years than the global average and 5.2 more years than men in the United States. When a team of 500 researchers from more than 300 institutions in 50 countries combined all their longevity data, Icelandic men outlasted all others.

The answer isn't likely cultural. Iceland's healthcare system is nothing special; most rankings don't list it as a standout. Its people aren't exactly runway models; they fall in the middle of the pack for obesity rates. They are in fact heavy eaters, consuming an average of 3,260 calories a day and eating fewer fruits and vegetables compared to other European countries. And there's no strong evidence indicating that Icelanders are more active than most other nations. Stefansson believes Icelandic longevity may have something to do with the story of its people.

In the year 874, the Vikings of northern Norway were sick of a quarrelsome king from the south who had taken over the country. So about 4,000 to 6,000 of the most pissed-off, risk-prone men in the north loaded themselves, sheep, cattle, and horses into Viking longboats and launched. They first sailed to the Shetland Islands and Ireland. There they kidnapped women (they were Vikings, after all), which grew their numbers to about 8,000. The Vikings then set back out into the North Atlantic, searching for a home.

This was no Carnival cruise. Viking longboats were narrow and light, with shallow hulls. Fast, but they could easily capsize in bad weather. And the advanced storm-warning techniques of the time mostly included praying and hoping.

But these Vikings were then the world's most advanced navigators. After a miserable five days at sea they found a destination. It was a patch of volcanic rock about the size of Kentucky that was covered in jagged rock, ice, and moss. It was constantly hit with wind, rain, snow, and cold. It was engulfed in darkness three-quarters of the year. It was devoid of edible life. It was now home. They called it Iceland.

A group of Celtic monks had once tried to live on the severe island. But they'd mysteriously vanished, never to be seen or heard from again.

Over the next 100 years, another 20,000 disaffected Norwegian men and kidnapped UK women arrived. All of these settlers quickly faced a jarring reality: "Iceland is a shit place to live," as one Icelander described it to me.

The most the settlers could grow was hay and grass, which they'd feed to sheep and cattle. So they ate sheep, cattle, and dairy products, and not a whole lot else. And there was never enough of that food.

The winters were nine months long. The country saw rain, hail, or snow 213 days a year. Winds regularly hit 40 miles an hour, sometimes reaching into the 100s.

The longest days in the dead of winter offered just four to five hours of dusky sunlight. As another Icelander explained to me, "In winter the sun comes up to say, 'Fuck you,' and then drops back down."

And that was just the everyday, uncomfortable white noise of living in Iceland. Sometimes the country pushed people over the edge.

"We know that living in this country for eleven hundred years has changed us, and we have evidence for that," said Stefansson while we drove the streets of Reykjavik in his black Porsche SUV. "In many ways, it's inevitable. Because humans are ultimately a consequence of a bunch of DNA macromolecules and the environment we live in."

It's the combination of DNA and environment—this formula of life and how we live in it—that determines our fate. Consider Julian and Adrian Riester, identical twins born in 1919. They had the same genetic code—and the same lifestyle, both becoming Catholic monks. They went to the same schools, ate the same meals, did the same tasks, etc. Their formula of life and living it were identical. They died of the same disease within hours of each other on June 8, 2011.

Discomfort is likely a key ingredient in the Icelandic formula, Stefansson was telling me. "It was never an easy time living here these eleven hundred years. There were volcanic eruptions. We lived in unheated houses for a thousand years in a very, very cold country. We had to earn a living by fishing in a rough sea. We faced infectious epidemics," Stefansson said, piloting the Porsche past Hallgrímskirkja, a towering stone cathedral that reaches into the turbulent Icelandic sky. "And so what has that done to us?" he asked.

It's a question that's long intrigued Stefansson as well as many others on the island. "Our history is characterized by many setbacks," Dr. Ottar Guðmundsson, an Icelandic historian, told me.

"Because of this harshness, there was no population increase here for many centuries," he said. In 1846, for example, Iceland logged the highest infant mortality rate ever recorded: 611 deaths per 1,000 births.

"It's almost as if the country put a limit on who could live here, and held us down in so many areas," said Guðmundsson. "But maybe this caused us to bloom in other areas."

Stefansson's unique background in complex genetic medicine has led him to try to figure out what makes Icelanders so durable.

He compared the DNA inside 1,100-year old skulls of the settlers of Iceland to the DNA of modern Icelanders and people living in northern Norway and the UK. "We found that the DNA from the settlers of Iceland is closer to the DNA of today's Norwegians and Celts than it is to the DNA of today's Icelanders," he said. Iceland, in other words, has radically changed its people.

Men from Norway and Ireland live roughly 79 years. Icelanders are now living anywhere from two to four years longer than the men of the countries from which the first Icelanders came.

And that's likely "a consequence of this merciless little island," said Stefansson. "This fucking wet rock in the North Atlantic that has been punishing us relentlessly for the last eleven hundred years." He pulled up to my hotel. "And this is not a superficial, esoteric statement."

Iceland's crucible of discomfort and disasters may have culled the herd. Natural selection suggests the people who couldn't hack it likely perished. Those with a high discomfort tolerance probably thrived. By happenstance, genetic drift (the term for random chance and catastrophic events leading to specific traits becoming more frequent in a population) would have altered the small, isolated country's gene pool in such a way that some ideal genes may have been given an opportunity to spread faster.

The result is that Icelanders may have buried within their genetic code a harder-to-kill gene, one that explains their longevity. If Stefansson can isolate this theoretical gene or set of genes, perhaps he and his team can figure out a way to bring it to the masses.

WHEN I ARRIVED HOME IN LAS VEGAS, I HAD TO IMMEDIATELY SHIFT BACK TO MODERN life and start chopping at all the work that had piled up over the weeks. I had classes to teach, an obnoxious amount of emails to respond to, and too many meetings to attend.

But about a month later a hundred pounds of frozen caribou meat shipped from the game butcher in Alaska arrived on my front porch and provided me with my first moments of reflection.

An audible sizzle filled the kitchen that evening as soft, ruby red backstraps hit a hot black cast-iron pan. Shimmering translucent blood (technically it's called myoglobin) dripped from one of the steaks, each drop flaring up as it touched the pan. I stared at the trickle, reminded of the lone stream of blood slowly falling from this very animal's neck as he lay on the Arctic tundra.

"What are you thinking about?" my wife asked. She was sitting at the kitchen island and answering emails on her laptop.

I looked over at her. "Do you think I've changed at all since I got back?" I asked.

"I think so," she said. "Since you've got back you're almost impossible to rattle. Nothing seems to bother you now."

Later that night I considered what she said. I surely felt different since my return. But I also knew I was affected by my past year digging into what we've lost with modern comforts.

Most obviously, I felt more aware. At a skin-deep level, this showed itself as a newfound appreciation for the incredible comforts of our modern world. My first week back I'd break out into an idiotic grin every time I turned on a faucet or drove a car or ate food that wasn't reconstituted sludge cooked and served in a plastic bag.

But on a deeper level I felt an awareness of time, how little of it we have, and what that can tell us about how we should use it. Marcus Elliott told me that a critical benefit of misogi is what he called "creating impressions in your scrapbook." "If you're seeing and doing all the same things over and over, your scrapbook looks pretty empty when you take inventory of your life," he said. "So we need to do more novel things to start creating more impressions in our scrapbooks, so we don't feel like the years are flying by. I mean, you remember every single detail of novel, meaningful experiences. You have no chance to forget them the rest of your life."

About a 19-mile, open-water Pacific Ocean swim misogi Nelson Parrish said, "As an artist, I thought I knew blue. But that misogi fully immersed me in so many shades, gradients, vibrancies, and transitions of blue. The water and sky. I now *know* blue. The experience drastically impacted my art, and I'll never forget those blues."

The difficulty and new challenges in Alaska left me with a massive new file of memories to relive and stories to tell. I'd experienced firsthand the phenomenon first theorized by William James and proven by recent studies, which shows that new events decelerate our perception of time.

I found myself applying these two lessons to my everyday life. I was thinking less and noticing more. I sought more connection, silence, and solitude both at home and in nature. I spent less time in front of screeens and was more of an active listener in conversations with my wife and family. At least twice a week I'd do a ruck in the desert and find a sort of sustained Zen traveling across the miles of red-rock-and-cactus-flanked trails. And my wife was right: I could see that my modern "problems" weren't real problems, so I was harder to rattle. Chasing that which makes humans harder to kill was, it seemed, making it easier for me to live.

In sobriety there's something called the "pink cloud" phenomenon. It describes the intense feelings of awareness, euphoria, connectedness, confidence, and calmness that occur in the early stages of recovery, right after a person has gone through the most uncomfortable phases of drying out. We realize we've pulled ourselves out of a slow death and become eager to *live*.

But the pink cloud eventually fades and real life sets in, leading many people to see if higher relief was in the bottle after all. My own pink cloud lasted about two years, until normalcy set in. I didn't fall off the wagon, but I did become somewhat restless and discontented.

Back from misogi, I felt like I was back on the pink cloud. Alaska provided me with another heavy dose of discomfort, and its lessons changed me. But I also understood that they wouldn't be everlasting, that comfort creep would gain inches each day. I'm already planning the next misogi.

I'm also now finishing this book in the midst of a global pandemic during which few would argue that they feel overly "comfortable." Too many have died, many more have been seriously ill, and millions beyond that have lost their livelihoods. But just as the pandemic forced nature itself to experience a sort of rewilding, from the cleaner canals of Venice to coyotes roaming around the mostly empty Golden Gate Bridge, we all did, too. It was a reminder that we're all still deeply connected to the natural world and that our technological advancements can't fix everything immediately. But it was also a rare break from the predictable. A moment for reflection, re-prioritizing, and maybe change.

ACKNOWLEDGMENTS

First and foremost, thanks to Leah, for all of her help, positivity, and support. She was the only person to read chapters and sections of this book and tell me "This is boring." She pushed me out of my comfort zone, and for that the work is better.

Thanks to my mom, a single parent and badass who played the role of mother and father and encouraged me to pursue writing.

Thanks to Matthew Benjamin, who edited this book and displayed an incredible eye for finding what matters. He found the best sentences and ideas buried within the rambling streams of consciousness I sent him, and he managed to turn them into something publishable.

Thanks to my literary agents, Jan Baumer and Steve Troha, who early in the process of developing the idea that would become this book asked "What happened to you?" and forced me to tell a truer story.

Thanks to Donnie, for so graciously allowing me to join him on such an epic adventure. It changed my life. I'm looking forward to the next one.

Thanks to the publications that let me use and adapt past materials for this book. Thanks, also, to my editors and mentors at those publications who shaped those stories and, in turn, this book. Especially Ben Court, Adam Campbell, and Bill Stump.

Thanks to all the sources in this book—particularly Trevor Kashey (x10), Marcus Elliott, Rachel Hopman, Karma Ura, Jason McCarthy, Kari Stefansson, Doug Kechijian, T.C. Worley, and Daniel Lieberman—who put up with my incessant questioning and naïveté and were so gracious with their time, wisdom, and patience.

Thanks to Kevin Stoker and Rob Ulmer in the Greenspun College of Urban Affairs at UNLV for being so supportive of this project.

Finally, thanks to Bill, for keeping me honest, willing, and accepting.

AUTHOR'S NOTE

This book developed in part from various articles I wrote for *Men's Health, Outside,* and *Vice.* Certain brief sections of those pieces appear nearly unaltered in this work.

In September and October 2019, I spent five weeks in Alaska, most of them deep in its backcountry. We traveled beyond the Arctic, but for the sake of clarity and narrative I have condensed the timeline in this book to include only our time in the Arctic.

I conducted many interviews and read hundreds of academic studies and lay materials in the process of reporting this book. Publishers maintain strict page-count limits, and instead of ceding valuable story and information to sourcing pages, I elected to put all source material online. For those interested, I have included references on every source in this book at eastermichael.com/tccsources.

INDEX

ABOUT THE AUTHOR

Michael Easter is a contributing editor at *Men's Health* magazine, columnist for *Outside* magazine, and professor at the University of Nevada, Las Vegas (UNLV). His work has appeared in more than 60 countries and can also be found in *Men's Journal, New York, Vice, Scientific American, Esquire,* and others. He lives in Las Vegas on the edge of the desert with his wife and their two dogs. For resources related to this book, such as the training program he used to prepare for Alaska and a list of the outdoor gear he used there, as well as other information applicable to misogi—plus new findings on the benefits of discomfort—check out Michael's website at eastermichael.com.